Atlas of Ambulatory EEG

Atlas of Ambulatory EEG

Editors

Bernard S. Chang, M.D.
Comprehensive Epilepsy Center
Beth Israel Deaconess Medical Center
Boston, Massachusetts

Steven C. Schachter, M.D.
Comprehensive Epilepsy Center
Beth Israel Deaconess Medical Center
Boston, Massachusetts

Donald L. Schomer, M.D.
Comprehensive Epilepsy Center
Beth Israel Deaconess Medical Center
Boston, Massachusetts

ELSEVIER
ACADEMIC
PRESS

Amsterdam Boston Heidelberg London New York Oxford
Paris San Diego San Francisco Singapore Sydney Tokyo

Elsevier Academic Press
30 Corporate Drive, Suite 400, Burlington, MA 01803, USA
525 B Street, Suite 1900, San Diego, California 92101-4495, USA
84 Theobald's Road, London WC1X 8RR, UK

This book is printed on acid-free paper. ♾

Library of Congress Cataloging-in-Publication Data

British Library Cataloguing in Publication Data
A catalogue record for this book is available from the British Library

ISBN 13: 978-0-12-621345-4
ISBN 10: 0-12-621345-3

For all information on all Elsevier Academic Press publications visit our Web site at www.books.elsevier.com

Printed in the United States of America
05 06 07 08 09 10 9 8 7 6 5 4 3 2 1

To Amanda and Benjamin (B.S.C.)

To Sue, Michael and David (S.C.S.)

To Peter Gloor, mentor and friend (D.L.S.)

Contents

Acknowledgments

The authors gratefully acknowledge SleepMed for providing EEG tracings.

Contributors

Frank W. Drislane, M.D.
Comprehensive Epilepsy Center
Beth Israel Deaconess Medical Center
Boston, Massachusetts

John R. Ives, B.Sc.
Department of Clinical Neurological Sciences
University of Western Ontario
London, Ontario, Canada

K. B. Krishnamurthy, M.D.
Comprehensive Epilepsy Center
Beth Israel Deaconess Medical Center
Boston, Massachusetts

Introduction

In the past few decades, ambulatory EEG has evolved from its inception as a novelty of clinical neurophysiology engineering to its current mature form as a routine clinical test ordered at local laboratories by neurologists worldwide. The rapid pace at which the technology, availability, and clinical utility of ambulatory EEG have advanced during this time has required electroencephalographers to keep up with the capabilities of this recording technique at an impressive rate.

Over this same time period the clinical neurophysiology world, of which ambulatory EEG is just one part, has been transformed. The development of specialized epilepsy centers has revolutionized the diagnosis and management of seizure disorders and brought focus to the need for prolonged EEG recording of high quality. In particular, the advent of epilepsy surgery as a major treatment option for some patients with medically refractory seizures has propelled the field of EEG monitoring forward. In addition, the increasing recognition of disorders that mimic epilepsy, including both psychogenic nonepileptic seizures (PNES) and physiological paroxysmal episodes that are nonepileptic, has also widened the spectrum of patients for whom EEG monitoring is appropriate.

However, financial and other constraints have affected the clinical use of neurophysiological studies to a significant degree. Physicians who are planning long hospitalizations for inpatient EEG recording must face the pressures of decreasing reimbursement, hospital space constraints, and patient dissatisfaction with in-hospital care. As the acuity of most hospitalized patients rises, so does the disparity between the typical neurology inpatient and the elective EEG-monitoring patient who has infrequent spells that may or may not be epileptic seizures.

Ambulatory EEG thus occupies an important niche in the clinical neurophysiology laboratory. Many patients who require prolonged EEG recording with event detection algorithms need not be admitted to the hospital; in fact both doctor and patient may prefer recording at home for convenience, the ability to capture events in the patient's natural environment, and the avoidance of inpatient nosocomial infection risk, among many other factors. The assumed sacrifice in recording quality that accompanied ambulatory EEG in its early days is now generally minimal or nonexistent, and the full extent of video recording and associated physiological parameter monitoring is now available on an ambulatory basis at many centers.

In this context, the clinical utility of an atlas of ambulatory EEG is clear. Although the principles of EEG interpretation remain unchanged regardless of recording environment, we believe that the ability of an electroencephalographer to review instructive examples of both normal and abnormal EEG activity recorded on an ambulatory basis will be significantly beneficial. Reference examples of common artifacts seen on ambulatory EEG and ictal events recorded using ambulatory systems may be particularly useful.

The three chapters in this book help to set the stage for the collection of ambulatory EEG excerpts and annotations presented later. In Chapter 1, John Ives and Don Schomer relate a brief history of ambulatory EEG technology from its inception to the present. Chapter 2, by K. Babu Krishnamurthy, describes the event-detection algorithms—both spike and seizure detection—that have facilitated the widespread use and interpretation of ambulatory EEG. Finally, in Chapter 3, Frank Drislane discusses the clinical role of ambulatory EEG in modern day epilepsy practice. The atlas figures that follow comprise those most likely to be of use to the practicing electroencephalographer, and are divided into examples of technical aspects, normal sleep morphologies, ambulatory artifacts, and abnormal epileptiform activity.

We believe our book will serve as a useful reference for a wide range of clinical neurophysiology practitioners, from trainees to experienced EEG readers, as well as for EEG technologists and others involved in the development and application of EEG recording software and hardware. After 30 years, countless innovations, and thousands of patient studies, ambulatory EEG now has its own atlas.

Bernard S. Chang
Steven C. Schachter
Donald L. Schomer
Boston, Massachusetts
July 2005

CHAPTER 1

A Brief History of Ambulatory EEG

JOHN R. IVES AND DONALD L. SCHOMER

I. Introduction

The first patient with epilepsy to be sent home with an ambulatory electroencephalogram (EEG) cassette recorder was evaluated at the Montreal Neurological Institute in the fall of 1973. [1, 2] Wearing a continuous recording, 4-channel, 24-hour device, he went downhill skiing. Later playback of that EEG (electroencephalogram) revealed several bursts of spike-and-wave discharges during that activity.

In the late 1980s, a patient with refractory seizures who was under consideration for epilepsy surgery was sent home from the Beth Israel Deaconess Medical Center, Boston, wearing a 27-channel event type ambulatory EEG recorder. The patient carried a solid-state small, 6-pound portable computer/hard drive EEG data acquisition unit that was capable of automatically detecting and recording spikes, sharp waves, and electrographic seizures.

Between the seventies and eighties there had been a natural evolution in the field of ambulatory-home EEG monitoring. This trend has continued over the past 15 years. Now, the use of ambulatory EEG monitoring for the diagnosis of patients with seizures, sleep disorders, and difficult-to-diagnose episodic events is common.

This chapter reviews the history of technological achievements that have led to today's ambulatory EEG monitoring systems.

II. The Rationale for Ambulatory Monitoring

Long-term ambulatory EEG monitoring (LTAM) is an important tool in the investigation of patients with epilepsy or those patients where a differential diagnosis exists that includes epilepsy. [3–5] In particular, LTAM can determine whether there is an EEG correlate to a particular event experienced by a patient. The clinical strategy is to record spontaneous events, using as many EEG channels as is practical, to provide clinically meaningful electrophysiological information concerning the nature and possible location of the patient's problem. These findings aid in the diagnosis of the disorder, and hence contribute to the treatment program.

Routinely acquired EEG documents the patient's background rhythm obtained in a very controlled state. One may capture interictal epileptiform activity as well. Routine EEG, however, is limited in duration and therefore is unlikely to record ictal events. Before the advent of long-term EEG monitoring of any kind, a survey of a large group of patients with focal onset seizure disorders who were under investigation for surgery at the Montreal Neurological Institute revealed that fewer than 25% of them had experienced a seizure while undergoing routine or prolonged routine recordings. [3, 6] Although a detailed review was not done, it is reasonable to expect that some of the seizures were recorded using montages that were not designed for seizure localization. Furthermore, the EEG activity on a significant number of the recorded seizures was likely obliterated by movement artifact due to the long electrode leads that were used to connect the patient to the EEG amplifiers. Other ictal tracings were likely obscured by muscle artifact due to the open bandwidth (0.5 to 70 Hz) routinely used during standard recordings. Therefore, a conservative estimate would be that fewer than 1 in 10 surgical candidates in this study had a technically acceptable ictal recording obtained during routine EEG acquisition. Consequently, the overwhelming majority of patients prior to 1970 underwent cortical resections based, in part, on the location of interictal epileptiform abnormalities recorded during conventional EEG testing. By contrast, today, surgical planning is based on the results of digitally recorded seizures.

During the 1970s, the development of video technology allowed the patient's peri-ictal behavior to be captured and time-locked to the EEG. As a result of this enhancement, there was a steady increase in the number and utilization of inpatient long-term EEG and video monitoring units. The requirement for documented seizures with video display of the behavior as an essential part of a presurgical workup also increased. [7–14] Inpatient EEG monitoring units using 16 or more channels of EEG with simultaneous video/audio soon became the standard method for documenting these ictal events. However, this testing paradigm became expensive and labor intensive, thus limiting the absolute number of facilities that could offer these services and hence limiting the number of patients that could be evaluated.

Ambulatory EEG monitoring was initially slow to gain acceptance due primarily to the lack of continuous video monitoring, which was considered essential. The technology of the day was not readily adaptable to the home environment. However, clinicians felt that the EEG was the more useful of the two streams of data (EEG and video) in the diagnosis of patients with epilepsy. LTAM was then used to determine which patients were more appropriate for the costlier hospital-based intensive EEG with video recording. When patients who were initially studied with LTAM were then hospitalized for EEG/video monitoring, there was a greater likelihood of obtaining relevant diagnostic information than in patients who underwent inpatient evaluation only.

Besides the cost and resource concerns, LTAM proved to be far more convenient for most patients. In some centers, including our own, inpatient monitoring became primarily utilized for patients whose seizures could only be recorded in the setting of anticonvulsant drug withdrawal. It was also used when simultaneous video recording was essential for diagnosis or surgical evaluation or in the setting where invasive electrodes needed to be used.

III. Continuous versus Event/Intermittent Recording

Two distinct types of ambulatory recording systems evolved largely independently of each other. One system provides continuous recording of EEG activity and the other obtains intermittent recording of events/seizures (i.e., noncontinuous).

A. Continuous Ambulatory Cassette Recording [16, 17]

The continuous recorder had its beginnings in 1947 when Norman Holter demonstrated a single-channel, radio-telemetry system that he used to transmit ECG signals. [18] His cardiac rhythm monitoring needed only a single channel of recording, which led to the development of the "Holter-type" electrocardiogram (ECG) monitors. [18] However, because a single channel of EEG is not very useful clinically, application to the ambulatory evaluation of patients with epilepsy awaited further technical development. A 4-channel continuous cassette recorder [19] was introduced and was later expanded to 8 channels of recording in the early 1980s and then to 32 channels in the late 1990s. The initial 4- and 8-channel EEG systems were used by the British navy for sleep research on subjects in the Antarctic (personal communications, Oxford Medical Systems). With the addition of neck-mounted miniaturized preamplifiers, a clinically useful ambulatory EEG system became practical. [1, 2]

The continuous ambulatory EEG recorder is essentially an extension of the routine EEG. All EEG activity is recorded and stored for later playback and review. As the technology evolved, so did the playback, recovery, analysis, and extraction of relevant EEG data from the 24-hour recorder. Initially, the 24-hour tapes could be recorded and replayed at a slower speed to permit the EEG to be transcribed through a conventional EEG machine onto paper. [20] An ink-jet EEG machine with significantly better high-frequency responses (700 Hz) enabled the entire EEG to be written out in less than 30 minutes in a highly compressed fashion (e.g., 20 minutes per standard EEG page). Electrographic ictal events stood out and were easily identified by the characteristic high-amplitude signatures that appeared when compared to baseline activity. Alternatively, the EEG could be reviewed through auditory analysis. Electrographic seizure discharges, background EEG rhythms, muscle artifact, etc., all produce very distinct and identifiable sounds [3, 17, 21] when played back at high speeds. Additionally, the 24-hour EEG could be automatically scanned by off-line data analysis software for morphologically distinct events such as spikes and seizures. Video display of the rapid pagination of 4-channel EEG was also developed as an efficient analysis technique for continuous 24-hour EEG. [23]

The advantage to the continuous recording methodology is that all of the EEG is recorded for an entire 24-hour period. This is useful when evaluating patients who have little to no advance warning of an impending seizure, such as patients with absence seizures. Electrographic seizures during sleep can also be identified. Having continuous EEG recording during sleep increases the probability of detecting interictal epileptiform activity in patients who do not have seizures during the daytime while being monitored. This may help to support a diagnosis of epilepsy.

Continuous EEG monitoring is also more appropriate for studies that quantify the number or duration of spike-wave paroxysms over a period of time. The video/audio replay technology of the day allowed the user to quickly identify the relevant EEG waveforms and to then review them visually via a variety of viewing systems. Continuous EEG recording was also necessary for most sleep evaluations, particularly if identification and characterization of sleep architecture was considered important.

The disadvantage of continuous ambulatory EEG monitoring, until recently, was the limited number of channels (4 or 8). This precluded detailed topographic characterization of abnormalities. Additionally, reviewers needed to be very experienced in order to play back the data in a way that was cost-effective.

Newer technological developments have eliminated the problems noted above. In the mid-1980s, a continuous 8-channel ambulatory system was introduced, followed by 16+ channel systems. A number of analysis features were added including digital, real-time automatic search capabilities based on either a specific time or an event marker. The new display included over a minute of data so that approximately 30 seconds before and after the "event" were presented on the screen. Gain and filter adjustments could be done on the screen without tape movement. Printout of the EEG, as displayed on the screen, was also possible. These new systems were able to record other forms of polygraphic data such as eye movement, muscle activity, cardiogram, and respiration, and opened the way for additional investigation. These advances allowed for testing other diagnostic disorders such as disordered cardiac rhythms or disordered sleep that may present as seizure-like behavior.

B. Event Type Ambulatory Cassette Recording

In the early 1970s, it was clear that obtaining weeks of continuous, paper-recorded EEG from inpatients undergoing depth electrode evaluations was unmanageable and overwhelming. Because the objective was to record the EEG during habitual seizures in these patients, the first step toward a rational solution was to develop a telemetry system that allowed patients to have some degree of freedom of movement during their hospitalization while recording their EEG rhythms. A system including on-the-head mounted amplifiers of the EEG-derived signal permitted this freedom. Artifact was significantly reduced using this "close to the source" amplification concept due to the lack of movement-related artifacts that are seen when recording with long electrode leads. The EEG signals were multiplexed, so 16 channels of EEG could be transmitted via a small wire to a DEC PDP-12 computer. A two-minute delay in the 16 channels of EEG was created by programming the digital computer to store EEG from the previous two minutes in a memory loop (i.e., buffering). This allowed the clinician to capture the onset of a clinical event even soon after it was in progress. [24] This started the era of EEG data manipulation and reduction.

Eventually, this loop concept was closed by including output software that reassembled the delayed EEG into the multiplexed format for transmission to another demultiplexing unit that was coupled to a Mingograph EEG machine. If a clinical event occurred, the activation of the seizure button caused it to be permanently stored on the computer tape. It also signaled the EEG machine to write out the two minutes of delayed EEG leading up to the event. The EEG machine was also programmed to take regular samples during the night in order to capture the natural sleep of the patient. [25]

As smaller microcomputers and larger memory systems became available, a stand-alone system was developed that could be moved to the patient's bedside. [26] This system consisted of an Intel 8085 computer with 1 Mbyte of RAM, an A/D-D/A input/output board, and a standard cassette tape deck to record the stored data. This unit emulated previous concepts that were on the larger computer, i.e., a delay loop with multiple multiplexed channels. A timecode generator was later added and this allowed independently recorded video to be synchronized to the EEG. [27] An EEG sample control unit automatically saved timed EEG samples at preset intervals, which allowed the clinician to see pieces of the patient's routinely generated EEG.

In the early 1980s, further electronic miniaturization enabled the functions of this bedside system to fit into an ambulatory cassette recorder. This "Walkman" audiocassette recorder stored the multiplexed EEG signals and the time-of-day signal. [28]. Initially, a number of technological constraints—power consumption, limited by the availability of static RAM—allowed for only a 5-second delay on the EEG. However, advancements in the field of SRAM memory circuits allowed two or more minutes of delay to be archived on ambulatory units. It also became possible to increase the channel capacity from 16 to 24 channels. [29] Thus, all major head regions could be covered simultaneously, including the use of sphenoidal electrodes. [30–32]

During a seizure, high-frequency muscle artifact can completely obscure the underlying EEG. A variety of filtering techniques have been developed in both digital [33] and analog [34] formats. Technical developments in the field of charge-coupled capacitive filters provided a simple and inexpensive means of replaying events that have been contaminated by high-frequency muscle artifact using a 6-pole filter with variable frequency settings ranging from 9 to 70 Hz. [35] This allows the clinician to replay events with a relatively open setting and compare that recording to playbacks with more extreme filtering and to note rhythms that are suspicious for seizure events.

Finally, a "time-scribe" digital clock capable of both displaying replay time and writing it out in a readable fashion on the EEG paper was developed to aid the time-locking of EEG with video, computer, or observation. [36, 37]

There were numerous advantages to the early periodic/event system. A greater number of recording channels was possible, which resulted in greater spatial resolution on recorded events. Patients and observers aided the EEG reader by selecting times of greater interest by pushing an event button when symptoms were experienced or clinical signs were observed. This also meant that there was less data to review. These systems were considerably less expensive than continuous recorders. The computer used for the automatic detection of relevant electrographic events could also be used to aid in the off-line analysis of a study.

There were also several disadvantages to the early intermittent ambulatory EEG recorders. There was dependence on an independent observer or the patient to know when a seizure was coming so the event button could be pushed. Also, the clinician could not go back and look at data prior to the delay time in cases where the event had a longer lead into it.

IV. Clinical Application

The continuous 4- and 8-channel systems and the event/periodic 16- and 24-channel systems have been used extensively in a variety of clinical settings. [16, 17] Their utility continues to expand as the technology of the systems matures and researchers define appropriate use. An example of this expanding role is the use of the 8-channel continuous system in polysomnography. [38, 39] The technological expansion from four to eight channels did not mean that the 4-channel systems were obsolete. It remains an ideal and useful 24-hour monitoring system for patients with spike-and-wave EEG abnormalities, especially if the goal is to determine the number or duration of discharges over a specific period of time.

In our center, all long-term monitoring is performed using the ambulatory systems. The degree of physical freedom for the patient depends on the clinical applications. In the outpatient environment, the patient may be sent home wearing the 16- or 24-channel ambulatory recorder and carrying a small event detection computer that is connected to the patient once they arrive at their home. In our hospitalized patient population, the recording options also depend upon the clinical situation. One option is to have the patient wear the 16- or 24-channel event recorder. This is done when the patient wants to go for a short walk or needs to be in another part of the hospital for other tests. When the patient is in their hospital room, they are plugged into a recorder via a telephone jack that connects the event detection computer to the patient and synchronizes the EEG signal to the continuous video recording.

By incorporating sleep montages into the ambulatory digital system and coupling this system with various other physiological recorders such as a portable SpO_2 sensor, one can perform ambulatory sleep recordings. The integration of an SpO_2 measuring transducer into the bedside EEG data acquisition device enables SpO_2 to be obtained simultaneously with EEG during seizures or during sleep. [40] One can now measure the depth of a hypopnea related to a stage of sleep or look for apnea during seizures. The recent introduction of a completely integrated, small, portable, and reliable home video/EEG recording system has addressed one of the last technical barriers for monitoring in the home. Now it is possible to obtain full EEG/video monitoring in the home environment.

There have been several additional advances in ambulatory EEG recording worth noting. [41] Continued development of digital storage devices has allowed the two fields of ambulatory monitoring to merge. One can now easily and conveniently record either continuous or intermittent data. The potential number of channels available for data has expanded to more than 128. The EEG activity can be easily remontaged so that events can be viewed with full remontage capability. Data transmission can be accomplished via a high-speed Internet link. This is more conducive to recording in outlying clinics or hospitals that are linked to a centralized site through a high-speed Internet link rather than to recording in the home environment, however. The video recordings are now all in digital formats, which allows for close-ups or wide angle viewing and high-resolution or low-light recordings. Additional sensors are being modified and adapted to run on low-power ambulatory systems that can be easily linked to the home recording platform.

V. Summary

As ambulatory EEG technology has become more of a routine and clinically established tool, its integration into the diagnostic evaluation of patients with possible or definite epilepsy is more widely accepted. At our center, for example, 30% of all EEG studies involve some ambulatory home monitoring. It seems likely that systems will continue to evolve and combine the best qualities of the continuous and event recorders. Ideally, these hybrid systems will replace both the current continuous recording systems and the event recorders. We are now looking forward to the 21st century where new developments may allow us to predict seizures and react to that information therapeutically.

References

1. Ives J. R., Woods J. F. 4-channel 24-hour cassette recorder for long term EEG monitoring of ambulatory patients. *Electroenceph. Clin. Neurophysiol.* 1975; 39:88–92.
2. Ives J. R. Electroencephalogram monitoring of ambulatory epileptic patients. *Postgrad. Med. J.* 1976; 52 (Suppl. 7):86–91.
3. Ives J. R., Woods J. F. The contribution of ambulatory EEG to the management of epileptic patients. In: *Clinical Ambulatory Monitoring*, Littler, W. A., ed. London: Chapman and Hall, 1980; 122–147.
4. Gotman J., Ives J. R., Gloor P., eds. *Long-Term Monitoring in Epilepsy* (EEG Suppl. No 37), Amsterdam: Elsevier Science Publishers BV, Biomedical Division, 1985.
5. Gumnit R. J., ed. *Intensive Neurodiagnostic Monitoring, Advances in Neurology,* Vol. 46, New York: Raven Press, 1987.
6. Rasmussen T. Localization aspects of epileptic seizure phenomena. In: *New Perspectives in Cerebral Localization*, Thompson R. A., Green J. R., eds. New York: Raven Press, 1982; 177–203.
7. Gotman J., Ives J. R., Gloor P., Quesney L. F., Bergsma P. Monitoring at the Montreal Neurological Institute. In: *Long-Term Monitoring in Epilepsy* (EEG Suppl. No 37), Gotman J., Ives J. R., Gloor P., eds. Amsterdam: Elsevier Science Publishers BV, Biomedical Division, 1985; 327–340.
8. Binnie C. D., Aarts J. H. P., Van Bentum-De Boer P. T. E., Wisman T. Monitoring at the Instituut voor Epilepsiebestrijding Meer en Bosch. In: *Long-Term Monitoring in Epilepsy* (EEG Suppl. No 37), Gotman J., Ives J. R., Gloor P., eds. Amsterdam: Elsevier Science Publishers BV, Biomedical Division, 1985; 341–356.
9. Ebersole J. S., Mattson R. H., Williamson P. D., Spencer S. S., Glaser G. H. Monitoring at the West Haven VA/Yale University School of Medicine Epilepsy Center. In: *Long-Term Monitoring in Epilepsy* (EEG Suppl. No 37), Gotman J., Ives J. R., Gloor P., eds. Amsterdam: Elsevier Science Publishers BV, Biomedical Division, 1985; 357–370.
10. Egli M., O'Kane M., Mothersill I., O'Kane F., Rai V. P. Monitoring at the Swiss Epilepsy Center. In: *Long-Term Monitoring in Epilepsy* (EEG Suppl. No 37), Gotman J., Ives J. R., Gloor P., eds. Amsterdam: Elsevier Science Publishers BV, Biomedical Division, 1985; 371–384.
11. Nuwer M. R., Engel J. Jr., Sutherling W. W., Babb T. L. Monitoring at the University of California, Los Angeles. In: *Long-Term Monitoring in Epilepsy* (EEG Suppl. No 37), Gotman J., Ives J. R., Gloor P., eds. Amsterdam: Elsevier Science Publishers BV, Biomedical Division, 1985; 371–384.

12. Kellaway P., Frost J. D. Jr. Monitoring at the Baylor College of Medicine, Houston. In: *Long-Term Monitoring in Epilepsy* (EEG Suppl. No 37), Gotman J., Ives J. R., Gloor P., eds. Amsterdam: Elsevier Science Publishers BV, Biomedical Division, 1985; 403–414.
13. Sato S., Long R. L., Porter R. J. Monitoring at the National Institute of Neurological Communicative Disorders and Stroke. In: *Long-Term Monitoring in Epilepsy* (EEG Suppl. No 37), Gotman J., Ives J. R., Gloor P., eds. Amsterdam: Elsevier Science Publishers BV, Biomedical Division, 1985; 415–422.
14. Roberts R., Fitch P. Monitoring at the National Hospital, Queen Square, London. In: *Long-Term Monitoring in Epilepsy* (EEG Suppl. No 37), Gotman J., Ives J. R., Gloor P., eds. Amsterdam: Elsevier Science Publishers BV, Biomedical Division, 1985; 423–436.
15. Riley T. L., Porter R. J., White B. G., Penry J. K. The hospital experience and seizure control. *Neurology (Cleveland)* 1981; 31:912–915.
16. Ebersole J. S. Ambulatory cassette EEG. *J. Clin. Neurophysiol.* 1985; 2(4):397–418.
17. Ebersole J. S., Bridges S. L. Ambulatory EEG monitoring. In: *Recent Advances in Epilepsy No. 3*, Pedley T. A., Meldrum B. S., eds. Edinburgh: Churchill Livingston, 1986; 111–135.
18. Holter N. J. New method for heart studies. *Science* 1961; 134:1214–1220.
19. Marson G. B., McKinnon J. B. A miniature tape recorder for many applications. *Control Instrum.* 1972; 4:46–47.
20. Wilkinson R. T., Mullaney D. Electroencephalogram recording of sleep in the home. *Postgrad. Med. J.* 1976; 52 (Suppl. 7):92–96.
21. Stalberg E. Experience with long-term telemetry in routine diagnostic work. In: *Quantitative Analytic Studies in Epilepsy*, Kellaway P., Petersen I., eds. New York: Raven Press, 1976; 269–278.
22. Quy R. J. A miniature preamplifier for ambulatory monitoring of the electroencephalogram. *J. Physiol. (London)* 1978; 284:23–24.
23. Stores G., Hennion T., Quy R. J. EEG ambulatory monitoring system with visual playback display. In: *Advances in Epileptology*, Woods J. A., Penry J. K., eds. The Xth Epilepsy International Symposium, New York: Raven Press, 1980; 89–94.
24. Ives J. R., Thompson C. J., Gloor P. Seizure monitoring: A new tool in electroencephalography. *Electroenceph. Clin. Neurophysiol.* 1976; 41:422–427.
25. Ives J. R., Gloor P. Automatic nocturnal sleep sampling: A useful method in clinical electroencephalography. *Electroenceph. Clin. Neurophysiol.* 1977; 43:880–884.
26. Ives J. R. "F4-P4": A self-contained mobile 16-channel EEG data acquisition system for recording seizures. *Electroenceph. Clin. Neurophysiol.* 1982; 54:37p.
27. Ives, J. R., Gloor P. A long-term time-lapse video system to document the patient's spontaneous clinical seizures synchronized with the EEG. *Electroenceph. Clin. Neurophysiol.* 1978; 45:412.
28. Ives J. R. A completely ambulatory 16-channel recording system. In: *Mobile Long-Term EEG Monitoring*, Stefan H., Burr W., eds. Stuttgard: Gustav Fischer, 1982; 205–217.
29. Ives J. R., Schomer D. L. Recent technical advances in long-term ambulatory outpatient monitoring. *Electroenceph. Clin. Neurophysiol.* 1986; 64:37p.
30. Ives J. R., Gloor P. New sphenoidal electrode assembly to permit long-term monitoring of the patient's ictal or interictal EEG. *Electroenceph. Clin. Neurophysiol.* 1977; 46:575–580.
31. Ives J. R., Gloor P. Update: Chronic sphenoidal electrode. *Electroenceph. Clin. Neurophysiol.* 1978; 44:789–790.
32. Ives J. R., Schomer D. L. The significance of using chronic sphenoidal electrodes during the recording of spontaneous ictal events in patients suspected of having temporal lobe seizures. *Electroencephal. Clin. Neurophysiol.* 1986; 64:23p.
33. Gotman J., Ives J. R., Gloor P. Frequency content of EEG and EMG at seizure onset: Possibility of removal of EMG artifact by digital filtering. *Electroenceph. Clin. Neurophysiol.* 1981; 52:626–639.
34. Barlow J. S. EMG artifact minimization during clinical EEG recordings by special analog filters. *Electroenceph. Clin. Neurophysiol.* 1984; 58:161–174.
35. Ives J. R., Schomer D. L. A 6-pole filter for improving the readability of muscle contaminated EEG. *Electroenceph. Clin. Neurophysiol.* 1988; 69:486–490.
36. Ives J. R. "Time-scribe": A universal time writer for any EEG/polygraph chart recorder. *Electroenceph. Clin. Neurophysiol.* 1984; 57:388–391.
37. Ives, J. R. Recording the time of day. *Long-Term Monitoring in Epilepsy* (EEG Suppl. No 37), Gotman J., Ives J. R., Gloor P., eds. Amsterdam: Elsevier Science Publishers BV, Biomedical Division, 1985; 83–89.
38. Wilkinson R. T., Mullaney D. Electroencephalogram recording of sleep in the home. *Postgrad. Med. J.* 1976; 52(7):92–96.

39. Hoelscher T. J., Erwin C. W., Marsh G. R., Webb M. D., Radtke A. A., Linnger A. Ambulatory sleep monitoring with the Oxford-Medilog 9000: Technical acceptability, patient acceptance, and clinical indications. *Sleep* 1987; 10:606–607.
40. Ives J. R., Mainwaring N. R., Krishnamurthy K. B., Blum A. S., Drislane F. W., Schachter S. C., Schomer D. L. Technical implementation and clinical findings/results of monitoring oxygen saturation in patients referred for long term EEG monitoring. *Electroenceph. Clin. Neurophysiol.* 1996; 99:432–439.
41. Schomer, D. L., Advances in EEG telemetry. In: *Advances in Clinical Neurophysiology 57*, Hallett, M., Phillips, L., Schomer, D. L., Massey K.M. eds. Amsterdam: Elsevier, 2005; 477–484.

CHAPTER 2

Automated Spike and Seizure Detection Algorithms

K. B. KRISHNAMURTHY

I. Introduction

The development and application of automated spike and seizure detection algorithms has revolutionized ambulatory electroencephalogram (EEG) monitoring. Initially, prolonged EEG monitoring was used to characterize the electrographic correlate of spells that were detectable clinically. Therefore, in order for the monitoring to be successful, the events had to have a clinical manifestation that was identifiable either by the patient or by an observer. [1] Prior to the introduction of automatic detection, EEG monitoring could not identify subclinical events, i.e., events that were not reported by the patient or obvious to an observer. For this reason, the early versions of EEG monitoring devices recorded 24 hours of continuous data that were then manually reviewed by a technologist and electroencephalographer—a labor-intensive and time-consuming process. [1] Typically, a trained technologist performed the initial review by screening the 24 hours of data and isolating events of interest for the EEG reader to further scrutinize. Another approach was for the entire record to be reviewed at speeds of up to 60 times real time by the EEG reader. [1]

The addition of computer-assisted spike and seizure detection has permitted the identification of interictal epileptiform abnormalities or electrographic seizures that are present at any time during the monitoring session. Liporace et al. demonstrated the increase in detection of interictal epileptiform abnormalities as well as subclinical seizures using ambulatory EEG with automated spike and seizure detection algorithms over sleep-deprived EEG. [2] Another study performed using an ambulatory EEG system that included automated spike and seizure detection algorithms showed that the likelihood of these computerized algorithms alone detecting an abnormality was 26.2%. [3] Automated seizure detection is particularly useful for patients who are not able to report clinical events or for those in whom seizures are not readily apparent to observers (such as those that might occur during sleep). In these patient groups, the use of automated algorithms for seizure detection enables clinicians to identify subclinical seizures and seizures for which the patient is amnestic without the need for a technologist to review the patient's entire EEG record. The ability to perform the recordings with the patients in their usual surroundings also allows for an increased possibility of capturing relevant events at a lower cost than inpatient telemetry. [4]

II. Automatic Spike Detection

As in routine EEGs, the detection of interictal epileptiform activity by automatic detection algorithms supports the diagnosis of epilepsy. [1] Among patients with known epilepsy and interictal abnormalities, as few as 40% may have a clinical seizure recorded over 48 to 72 hours of EEG monitoring. Thus the presence of interictal abnormalities in some cases may be the only abnormality present that is consistent with a diagnosis of epilepsy. [5] Automatic spike detection greatly reduces the time necessary to detect interictal discharges; a few pages contain the findings of interest without the need to laboriously scan the entire EEG.

Rigorous mathematical equations that precisely detect spike and sharp waves have not been established. The general strategy behind spike or sharp wave detection algorithms is to identify false detections in preference to missing true epileptiform discharges. However, the presence of short duration artifacts can contaminate the record, so artifact-free portions of the recording must be used.

A. Spike Detection Algorithms

The spike detection algorithms often used in ambulatory EEG monitoring systems are based upon pattern recognition. Complex EEG signals are redefined by a series of simpler elements through a series of steps that address three specific characteristics of the wave in question.

The first characteristic is the relative amplitude of sequential half-waves. For this analysis, every channel of EEG is divided into a series of segments; each segment consists of a section of EEG between two extremes of amplitude, for example, between the most negative and most positive positions. Because low-amplitude, high-frequency activity (e.g., muscle activity) can falsely influence the determination of a segment, some algorithms use filtering to attenuate such activity.

The Gotman/Gloor spike detection algorithm is designed to recreate the slow frequency wave while "smoothing" out low-amplitude fast activity. [6] It does this by evaluating trends in the directions of amplitudes—small segments going in a direction opposite to the major direction of activity are eliminated. This essentially eliminates high-frequency, low-amplitude elements. Pairs of segments, sequences, or a segment and a sequence are then combined into waves. Each wave consists of two elements with opposite directions.

Defining the amplitude of a segment or sequence comprising a half-wave is the next step in spike detection. Because this amplitude can only be relative to the background, it is necessary to constantly have a fix on the EEG background amplitude. This background amplitude is calculated three times per second continuously as the average amplitude of the sequences from the preceding 5 seconds. Thus, the relative amplitude of a half-wave is the ratio of its absolute amplitude to the background amplitude rounded to the closest integer from 0 to 20.

Another characteristic that determines whether a wave will be identified as a spike is a measure of its sharpness. This is calculated as the relative second derivative of the apex of its wave, using a portion of the waveform that includes 15 msec before and 15 msec after the apex. The background amplitude for the preceding 5 seconds of signal is used as a normalization factor.

The third and final characteristic that is analyzed is the pseudo-duration of each half-wave. This pseudo-duration incorporates information about the convexity of the half-wave, which makes it easier to differentiate between half-waves that are more or less likely to be part of a spike or sharp wave. The pseudo-duration compares the convexity of the beginning portion of a segment to the convexity of the final portion, which is felt to be a more appropriate and efficient measure of the duration of a half-wave. [6]

The spike detection algorithm is then applied to each half-wave of each channel independently. The following conditions must be met in order to categorize a given wave as a spike or sharp wave.

1. The relative amplitude of the current and preceding half-waves must be above a preset threshold.
2. The pseudo-durations of the current and preceding half-waves must be under a preset limit.
3. The relative amplitude must be large enough given the relative sharpness of the half-wave.
4. The total duration of the wave must be greater than or equal to a preset minimum value.

If all four conditions are met, the wave is selected as a possible spike or sharp wave. If any condition is not met, the wave is eliminated from consideration as a spike or sharp wave.

This algorithm does not identify electromyography (EMG) activity as spikes, because EMG activity is of short duration or because dividing it into segments causes too many segments for the calculation procedure. Similarly, it rejects eye-blink artifact seen in a frontal channel if a similar wave occurs in the same channel on the contralateral side, if it has a duration greater than 150 msec and if it has positive polarity. Finally, sharp or suddenly appearing alpha rhythm will be rejected if the wave in question is determined to be part of a section with a dominant frequency of 8 to 12 Hz.

B. Validation

The absolute accuracy of a computerized detection method is difficult, if not impossible, to ascertain. It can only be compared with the "standard" method, i.e., human review of EEG data. As concordance between human reviewers can be quite low, the validity of comparing the outcome of any algorithm with the results of a group of human interpreters can be questioned. Ultimately, because the spikes identified by the computer algorithm are also checked for accuracy by human observers, the capability of the computer program to identify events of interest is most important.

Because of this, Gotman et al. undertook a two-part study. [7] Initially, information about the likelihood of false positive and false negative identifications by the automated detection system was obtained. Secondly, a direct comparison between epileptiform activity identified by the computer algorithm and that identified by human reviewers was made.

To do this study EEGs were obtained in 30 healthy subjects, 30 patients with supratentorial brain lesions but no epilepsy, and in 50 patients with epilepsy. Two to three minutes of EEG were obtained for each subject in the resting state with eyes closed.

All computer-detected events identified in records from normal subjects and those obtained in nonepileptic patients were reviewed to determine if the event was an artifact (e.g., EMG, sharp alpha, or eye blinks). There were 21 detections that were identified as artifacts.

It was assumed that any interictal spikes or sharp waves identified by the detection algorithm in EEGs of healthy subjects and nonepileptic patients had to be false detections; this assumption is reasonable based on normative studies. [8] Therefore, all events identified in the EEGs of these subjects were initially categorized as "clearly erroneous detections." Later, these detections were visually inspected to determine if they truly were erroneous. In addition, the events identified as epileptiform in patients with epilepsy that were artifactual from EMG activity, eye blinks, or sharp alpha activity were also characterized as clearly erroneous detections. For the remaining detections, namely those in EEGs from patients with epilepsy, two EEG readers independently reviewed the paper recordings and each event identified by the computer. They had no knowledge of which detection came from which patient and filled out questionnaires (called structured reports) that were then compared.

These comparisons demonstrated that 4 out of the 50 paper tracings from patients with epilepsy contained no spikes according to both EEG readers; the computer algorithm also found no epileptiform abnormalities. In one case, after reviewing a paper recording both EEG readers found "mild and doubtful" abnormalities, which the computer detection algorithm failed to identify.

In general, there was 58 to 61% correlation between the findings of the EEG reading by the EEG readers and the computer detection algorithm. There was a 72% correlation between the two EEG readers for paper recordings, and a remarkable 84% agreement between EEG readers for review of the events identified by the computerized spike detection algorithm. This study demonstrated that computerized data acquisition/spike detection may diminish the inter-observer variability that characterizes the interpretation of paper EEGs.

III. Seizure Detection

For a seizure detection algorithm to be useful it must have a low number of missed detections (false negatives). False positive detections are not bothersome unless a large number occur. [9] The difficulty, however, lies in the fact that electrographic seizures can have a variety of patterns and are therefore much less likely to be uniform. [10] Also, rhythmic artifacts that frequently occur, such as EMG or eye-blink artifact, can be identified as possible seizures by some seizure detection algorithms. [10]

The first attempt at such an algorithm was by Prior et al., who used the combination of EMG activity and change in EEG amplitude (initial large increase in amplitude followed by a clear decrease) to identify generalized tonic-clonic seizures. [10, 11] This method was not useful for other seizure patterns such as those characterized by an electrodecremental response.

A. Seizure Detection Algorithms

The Gotman algorithm for seizure detection is capable of recognizing seizures of different types as long as at least a part of the seizure contains sustained paroxysmal rhythmic activity of 3 to 20 Hz. There are five steps to this algorithm.

First, a digital filter is applied to remove 60-Hz contamination. Then, a 2-second segment of one channel of EEG data, referred to as an epoch, is broken down into half-waves, further eliminating low-amplitude fast frequency activity.

Next the average amplitude (to confirm that an epoch is paroxysmal), average duration (a measure of frequency), and coefficient of variation of duration of half-waves in one epoch are calculated. [10] The coefficient of variation is a measure of the rhythmicity of the EEG, independent of the frequency of the waves involved.

The average amplitude in the previous step is calculated based upon the difference from the "background." This background period is updated for each new epoch and is calculated as follows:

1. The current epoch lasts for 2 seconds.
2. A 12-second gap is left which ends at the beginning of the current epoch.

3. The background section is a 16-second period that ends at the beginning of the 12-second gap.

Finally, a seizure detection is made when two or more channel detections occur in the same or adjacent epochs. If the two channel detections are in the same epoch but in two different channels, the average amplitude of the successive epoch in one of the two channels must be at least 80% that of the detection epoch. A channel detection has to satisfy three conditions: the relative amplitude is greater than or equal to 3, the average duration of half-waves is between 25 and 150 msec, and the coefficient of variation of the half-wave duration is less than 0.6. Therefore, detections will be triggered by a sudden increase in frequency or by rhythmic activity of large amplitude. [10]

A sixth step is used for rejection of artifacts. EMG activity, when broken down into half-waves, typically causes more than 100 half-wave segments in an epoch; rejection of an epoch containing more than 100 segments eliminates this type of false detection. Also, an epoch containing large amplitude technical artifacts is rejected if the maximal allowable amplitude is detected over 30 sampled data points in a given epoch. The epoch prior to the epoch in question is also rejected. [9]

This algorithm detects the rhythmic or paroxysmal part of the electrographic seizure but not necessarily the onset. Systems with large, rewritable buffers overcome this problem because computerized detection of the event in question can include the previous 2 minutes of recording. [10]

B. Validation

Gotman studied 5303 hours of continuous EEG recordings obtained from 49 patients. These comprised 241 recordings from 44 patients using scalp and sphenoidal electrodes and 52 recordings from 5 patients using intracerebral electrodes. In this sample, 244 seizures were recorded of which 59 were detected clinically alone, 86 were detected both clinically and by the detection algorithm, and 99 seizures were detected by the algorithm alone. [12] This finding suggests that a combination of automated detection and clinical observation produces the best outcome in terms of seizure detection.

IV. Conclusion

Automated spike and seizure detection algorithms are clinically reliable methods of screening for epileptiform and electrographic seizure activity, and thereby enhance the usefulness of ambulatory EEG monitoring. These algorithms are robust, and when used in conjunction with review of clinically apparent events they increase the possibility of capturing an abnormality that could alter the patient's treatment.

References

1. Bridgers S. L., Ebersole J. S. Cassette electroencephalography. In: *The Treatment of Epilepsy: Principles and Practices*, E. Wyllie, ed. Philadelphia: Lea & Febiger, 1993; 278–284.
2. Liporace J., Tatum W., Morris G. L., French J. Clinical utility of sleep-deprived versus computer-assisted ambulatory 16-channel EEG in epilepsy patients: A multi-center study. *Epilepsy Res.* 1998; 32:357–362.
3. Morris G. L., Galezowska J., Leroy R., North R. The results of computer-assisted ambulatory 16-channel EEG. *Electroenceph. Clin. Neurophysiol.* 1994; 91(3):229–231.
4. Waterhouse E. New horizons in ambulatory electroencephalography. *IEEE Eng. Med. Biol.* 2003; May/June:74–80.
5. Ebersole J. S., Leroy R. F. An evaluation of ambulatory, cassette EEG monitoring: II. Detection of interictal abnormalities. *Neurology* 1983; 33:8–18.
6. Gotman J., Gloor P. Automatic recognition and quantification of interictal epileptic activity in the human scalp EEG. *Electroenceph. Clin. Neurophysiol.* 1976; 41:513–529.

7. Gotman J., Gloor P., Schaul N. Comparison of traditional reading of the EEG and automatic recognition of interictal epileptic activity. *Electroenceph. Clin. Neurophysiol.* 1978; 44:48–60.
8. Schachter S. C., Ito M., Wannamaker B. B. et al. Incidence of spikes and paroxysmal rhythmic events in overnight ambulatory computer-assisted EEGs of normal subjects: A multi-center study. *J. Clin. Neurophys.* 1998; 15:251–255.
9. Gotman J. Automatic recognition of epileptic seizures in the EEG. *Electroenceph. Clin. Neurophysiol.* 1982; 54:530–540.
10. Gotman J., Burgess R. C., Darcey T. M., Harner R. N., Ives J. R., Lesser R. P., Pign J. P. M., Velis D. Computer applications. In: *Surgical Treatment of the Epilepsies*, Engel, J. Jr., ed. New York: Raven Press, Ltd. 1993; 429–443.
11. Prior P. F., Virden R. S. M., Maynard D. E. An EEG device for monitoring seizure discharges. *Epilepsia* 1973; 14:367–372.
12. Gotman J. Automatic seizure detection: improvements and evaluation. *Electroenceph. Clin. Neurophysiol.* 1990; 76:317–324.

CHAPTER 3

The Clinical Use of Ambulatory EEG

FRANK W. DRISLANE

I. Purposes of EEG Monitoring

Electroencephalogram (EEG) monitoring of patients with seizures or seizure-like symptoms can serve several purposes. [1–3] This chapter focuses on event (such as seizure) monitoring, particularly in the ambulatory setting.

A. Diagnosis of Epilepsy

The most basic and probably the most common use of EEG monitoring is to determine whether a patient with paroxysmal clinical disturbances is having epileptic seizures. Monitoring can help both in identification of interictal epileptiform discharges and in recording clinical seizures or seizure-like events. It can help identify whether an individual episode in question is epileptic or nonepileptic in origin.

Logically, it is probably impossible to exclude an epileptic basis for a given event. Some seizures are not well recorded at the surface EEG leads. Nevertheless, maintenance of a normal EEG background (even amid extensive movement and other artifact) suggests strongly that the event is not epileptic. Even if epileptiform discharges are not seen during some true epileptic seizures, there is usually a substantial alteration in the EEG with seizures such as rhythmic slowing, background suppression, or some other change.

Some paroxysmal clinical episodes are associated with clear electrographic seizures, helping to make the diagnosis. The absence of epileptiform EEG abnormalities at the time of paroxysmal behavioral disturbances increases the likelihood that the events are not epileptic, but rather manifestations of other illnesses. Two other groups of illnesses produce symptoms similar to those of seizures. There are events of other physiologic bases such as cardiac arrhythmias causing syncope, episodes caused by cerebrovascular disease, movement disorders, and unusual manifestations of sleep disorders. There are also events of psychiatric origin. Taken together, all of these events are generally referred to as "nonepileptic seizures." All of these can produce bizarre and unusual movements and behavior with some resemblance to epileptic seizures.

For some events, review of a video recording alone is persuasive for a psychogenic origin of spells. Nevertheless, even very experienced epileptologists will see bizarre behavior that appears to be psychogenic but, by EEG, actually has an epileptic basis.

The events of psychiatric origin are often referred to as psychogenic nonepileptic seizures (PNES), or pseudo-seizures or nonepileptic events. (Although used often, the word seizure in this context is likely to promote confusion.) EEG monitoring, especially with simultaneous video recording, is particularly valuable in the evaluation of possible PNES. Although not always successful, it is usually the best way to determine the nature of these events.

Epileptic seizures and PNES differ in several respects. [4–6] PNES tend to be of longer duration and may peak in frequency early in a monitoring session, whereas epileptic seizures tend to occur later, as medication is reduced. Medication withdrawal does not appear to influence the occurrence of nonepileptic events. Whereas PNES tend to occur in the daytime and not during sleep, epileptic seizures are common in sleep. The presence of observers and family members may prompt the occurrence of nonepileptic events and facilitate their recording. Many other clinical features help to distinguish epileptic from psychogenic events. [5, 6] An accurate diagnosis of PNES can be just as helpful as a diagnosis of epilepsy, at least for avoiding anticonvulsant toxicity.

Ambulatory EEG has been very effective at separating seizures from PNES in children, especially when the events in question are stereotyped and reliably discerned by observers such as parents. In these cases, video recording is often unnecessary. [7] Still, events need to occur with a reasonable frequency (such as three times per week) for monitoring to be successful.

As with any other test the value and, in this case, specificity of monitoring depend on the appropriateness of the events being monitored. [8] Monitoring to confirm a clinical suspicion of epilepsy or analyze clinically diagnosed epilepsy has a far greater yield than monitoring for vague or poorly characterized symptoms. In almost all cases, however, the yield is far greater than with routine EEG recordings. Still, events can be missed, and if the events in question do not occur during the session, monitoring may yield no useful results.

B. Determining Seizure Types and Epilepsy Syndromes

Even if it is clear on clinical grounds that the symptoms of interest are actually epileptic seizures, it is important to determine the type or types of seizures a patient has. Characterization of ictal and interictal abnormalities can help to determine seizure types and epilepsy syndromes, in conjunction with other clinical features and family history. Even with an accurate diagnosis of epilepsy, it is often appropriate to determine whether new, additional, or different behavioral episodes are seizures or not—there could be both seizures and PNES. This may become pertinent when a patient's seizures are poorly controlled; it may be asked whether the original diagnosis is correct.

The EEG recorded at the time of an event can help in seizure and epilepsy classification. It is commonly difficult to determine clinically whether a patient has a primary generalized or focal (localization-related) epilepsy. The recording of generalized spike-wave discharges or focal abnormalities obtained interictally or, better, during seizures, can help to make this distinction. For example, a young adult may have staring spells that are clearly epileptic in origin, but the treatment and prognosis may differ depending on whether the spells are primary generalized "absence" seizures or focal-onset complex partial seizures.

C. Localization

One of the most common reasons for EEG monitoring is to localize seizure onset in the evaluation of a patient with refractory epilepsy who is considering surgery after medications have failed to control the seizures. Documentation of seizures and the localization of their onset are crucial in the evaluation of patients considered for epilepsy surgery. It must be certain that the operative target is responsible for the seizures actually troubling the patient rather than for electrographic seizures that may not have a clinical correlate.

This information must be used in concert with neuroimaging findings such as those on MRI scans (especially with gadolinium enhancement and on fluid attenuated inversion recovery sequences; FLAIR); by evidence of neuronal damage or dysfunction on magnetic resonance spectroscopy (MRS); foci seen with single photon emission computerized tomography (SPECT) scans, especially those done at the time of seizures ("ictal SPECT"); and results from positron emission tomography (PET) scans, which show areas of abnormal metabolism interictally in patients with seizure foci. The ictal EEG remains the cornerstone of localization in most epilepsy surgical centers. [9] Plans for surgery are more secure when at least several seizures have been recorded and there is reliable determination of a (preferably single, isolated) seizure focus. A complete review of the utility of ictal EEG monitoring in surgical planning is beyond the scope of this chapter.

D. Examination for Subclinical Seizures

Some seizures recorded during prolonged EEG monitoring may be asymptomatic or "subclinical." Many such seizures can occur during sleep and are not noted by patients or observers. Some patients whose seizures are thought to be under good control on medication actually have frequent subclinical seizures. It is unclear that these seizures are actually subclinical (i.e., such electrographic seizures may have some immediate or even long-term clinical consequence), but this is still controversial. Some neurologists feel it is important to look for brief subclinical seizures when tapering or changing anticonvulsants to see if the situation is becoming worse before longer and potentially harmful seizures are evident clinically.

E. Monitoring for Seizures in the Postictal Period

Following seizures or status epilepticus (SE), especially when mental status is still impaired, many patients to actually have seizures or SE that is not evident clinically. Several groups have found that about 10% of patients who were thought to have had seizures or SE treated successfully were still in non-convulsive status epilepticus (NCSE). [10] Even among comatose patients with no clinical seizures at all, 8% were in NCSE in one study. [11] SE in the ICU is usually not suspected [12]; this is often a serious condition that can be treated successfully—but not if it remains undiagnosed. [13]

F. Assessment of Seizure Frequency

A somewhat less common use of EEG monitoring is quantitation of seizure frequency when the clinical history is not sufficient (including when individual episodes are not clearly epileptic). This may be particularly helpful when the patient is unable to provide an adequate report or when those reports are unreliable. Occasionally, this quantitation can help in deciding whether to increase or decrease the dosages of medication treatment. Nevertheless, it is difficult to depend on the data from a few days' recording to assess the impact of different medications on longer term seizure control. Absence seizures in adolescence may be among the few seizures for which neurologists will want to increase anticonvulsant treatment for very frequent subclinical seizures, usually with the thought that the patient may still suffer true clinical deficits of which he is not aware or that there may be deleterious cognitive effects of having many seizures.

G. Other Uses

EEG monitoring acquires much more data than routine EEGs. It can be better in detecting interictal abnormalities, particularly in patients who have normal baseline EEGs or who have findings of questionable significance such as various sharp transients. Cardiac arrhythmias may also be found. Sleep disorders may be identified, particularly when eye movement, electromyography (EMG), and respiratory function are monitored in addition to the EEG recording of sleep states. Determination of the precipitants for seizures can also be detailed through monitoring, e.g.,in catamenial and reflex-related seizure disorders.

II. Event Monitoring

EEG monitoring can record interictal epileptiform discharges and other physiologic variables such as cardiac rate and rhythm, respiratory function in sleep testing, partial pressure of oxygen, EMG, and movement-related activity. Monitoring also includes prolonged recording of the EEG, even at times when the patient has no symptoms. It can include algorithm-based recording of EEG features of interest such as spikes and electrographic seizures (see Chapter 2). Automatic seizure detection programs are useful, especially for seizures that occur in certain situations such as during sleep—when neither the patient nor observers are able to identify them. Nevertheless, it is the monitoring of individual episodes or paroxysmal events of abnormal clinical behavior that usually bring the patient in for medical attention and are of greatest interest.

Seizures are paroxysmal electroclinical events. This leads to two problems in EEG monitoring. First, the events are not present all of the time. Indeed, they may occur for just a minute or less in a 24-hour period, and the rest of a day's recording may yield little diagnostic information. Consequently, one must know exactly when the event occurred, or monitor the entire day's EEG and then search through and analyze very large quantities of data, most of which is of little interest. Recording may be continuous, but it is necessary to have some event markers to determine which epochs are of clinical interest. Focusing on the symptoms that constitute the chief complaint is a more effective way to evaluate a patient's symptoms.

Second, the precise correlation of the clinical disturbance and the recorded EEG abnormalities are of interest to both the patient and the neurologist. There must be a connection between the electrographic abnormality and the symptoms that trouble the patient. Some EEG abnormalities may not disturb the patient at all while others may explain the chief complaint. The goal of event recording is to record the seizures that trouble a patient more than interictal abnormalities or subclinical seizures alone.

For demonstration of the epileptic nature of individual spells and for localization it is desirable to record more than one event. Just as patients may have more than one type of seizure, some may have both epileptic seizures and nonepileptic events within the same day. It must be clear that the symptom of interest has been recorded.

Event-triggered systems often include video recording, particularly in the inpatient setting and when EEG findings may be absent or difficult to interpret, e.g., with some seizures of frontal origin. Video monitoring can show behavioral manifestations strongly suggestive of seizures or of nonepileptic events, even when the EEG is inconclusive. Notation of the event's timing is important in determining which portion of a video recording to review.

The best recording of symptoms comes from the detailed report of a patient who is able to describe which symptoms are most troublesome and whether an individual event includes those symptoms. This is often effected through use of a pushbutton event marker denoting the time of the event or marking the EEG itself. This should be accompanied by a description of the symptoms in a log or by audio recording.

Many patients have seizures that interfere with their ability to record the event. For example, patients who have partial seizures that undergo rapid generalization may lose consciousness or progress into a confusional state, which renders them unable to activate the system or describe their symptoms at the time. For many seizures involving limbic structures, there is amnesia for the event. In these cases notation of the event by an observer, often using the same pushbutton event marker, is essential. Certainly, children and patients with mental retardation or other neurological deficits hindering their own participation will need assistance from observers, both in intensive inpatient monitoring units and during ambulatory recording.

Many event-centered monitoring technologies depend heavily on observers such as family members, friends, or clinical personnel. An advantage of family observers is that they are often very familiar with the typical spells of interest and can describe whether individual spells are those of concern or whether the events are different.

Observers must watch the patient carefully for staring spells, interruption of speech, change in level of consciousness, or any altered behavior. Because the beginnings of many seizures are subtle, observers must be attentive to the patient at all times, a requirement that is not satisfied easily. Frequent interaction with the patient can help to ascertain continued consciousness, attentiveness, and normal speech and behavior. Particularly with such interaction, observers may help to record seizures that would not otherwise be apparent to observers or to patients themselves. Seizures manifested by subjective sensations alone (without obvious alteration in alertness or behavior) remain unnoticed by observers unless the patient reports them.

For subclinical or electrographic seizures and for nocturnal recording, techniques other than pushbutton activations are required. These may include automated seizure detection programs. When events are recorded by patients or observers voluntarily and also by automatic computer detection algorithms, it becomes clear that the two methods are not equivalent. Some events labeled seizures by the electroencephalographer, after reviewing a change in the EEG along with suggestive video observations, may not be detected by a given computer algorithm. Correspondingly, some automated detection programs record presumed electrographic seizures that are clearly artifactual or definitely not felt to be epileptic when reviewed by the electroencephalographer.

There are disadvantages to focusing on events and event recordings. It may fail when the patient is unable to record symptoms, when symptoms or signs of seizures are not apparent to observers, when observers are inattentive, and when seizures are truly subclinical to both patients and observers. These events are unlikely to be recorded. Many truly epileptic seizures occur during sleep. Observers may notice seizures in sleep, but this depends on awake, attentive observers.

Symptomatic events appear to occur more frequently in patients with psychogenic seizures than in patients with seizures of epileptic origin. [4] In this sense, patients with PNES are particularly cooperative with monitoring. In this setting, event recording can also be aided by suggestion or reproduction of common precipitants. [14] Video recording of particularly bizarre and physiologically unlikely behavior, without EEG abnormalities or alterations in the EEG baseline, can be very helpful in suggesting the diagnosis of PNES.

III. Ambulatory EEG Monitoring

Inpatient monitoring often entails a long hospitalization and is resource-intense in terms of staffing, hospital facilities, and maintenance of a monitoring unit. Ambulatory monitoring has been developed over the past 20 years and is now comparably reliable to monitoring done in the hospital. [8, 15]

Inpatient monitoring is more expensive, but it is not always better. In many cases, ambulatory outpatient EEG monitoring may be preferable, especially when it does not require anticonvulsant reduction. Ambulatory monitoring allows patients more mobility and the possibility of remaining in their natural environments and maintaining their usual activity level. It is more desirable to know the frequency of seizures in the patient's natural setting than in the hospital. Ambulatory monitoring is particularly suitable for patients whose events are more likely to occur in a familiar setting. Specific environmental stimuli may precipitate a patient's seizures, and they may be more readily available at home. Seizures related to sleep (e.g., nocturnal seizures) may be particularly dependent on the usual, home environment. Many patients have a marked reduction in seizure frequency upon admission to a hospital, where it can take weeks for seizures to occur, even though they were happening daily at home. [16] This may result from more reliable medication administration in hospital or from the security or lack of the usual environmental precipitants. In most cases, ambulatory monitoring also requires observers who are usually family members.

When seizures are frequent and there is no need to withdraw anticonvulsants, ambulatory monitoring can even be of sufficient quality to serve surgical candidates. These are usually patients with temporal lobe seizures. One report of six patients demonstrated that ambulatory EEG seizure monitoring could be safe, convenient, and sufficiently effective to plan surgery for patients with refractory temporal lobe epilepsy, with surgical results similar to those for patients who had inpatient monitoring. [17] Patients had similar baseline seizure frequency, numbers of seizures recorded, and time required to record three seizures. They had no significant complications. It is not clear that such monitoring would be sufficient for patients with extratemporal foci with refractory seizures.

Use of video recording can limit ambulatory monitoring. Video recording of clinical events is frequently crucial, particularly in the determination of epilepsy versus psychogenic events. It necessitates keeping the patient in view of the camera, usually limiting freedom of movement. It is important to synchronize the video and EEG recordings so that they can be analyzed simultaneously. Outpatient video and EEG monitoring requires the patient or family to be comfortable enough with the technology to operate the equipment and be responsible for expensive monitoring equipment. Fortunately, such equipment has become much more simplified in its operations and even familiar to many non-medical people accustomed to consumer electronics. Increasingly, video recording can be synchronized with ambulatory EEG at home, but the quality is not always as good as in inpatient units. The cost savings of ambulatory monitoring must, of course, be balanced by a concern for patient safety (and equipment damage) if there are vigorous or violent convulsions in a less well-controlled setting.

Anticonvulsant medication reduction is used often to elicit events of clinical interest, with the potential risk of precipitating excessive seizures or even status epilepticus (SE). Therefore, the need to reduce anticonvulsant dosages necessitates hospital admission. Medication withdrawal must be performed carefully in patients with worrisome seizures. Even a minimal diminution of anticonvulsants can precipitate dangerous seizures or SE. One study indicated that 3% of patients with complex partial seizures monitored in epilepsy units went on to have SE despite close observation, and another 8% had clusters of at least three seizures in four hours. [18] Such clusters may be a precursor to SE, so detecting frequent seizures is usually considered important clinically. Also, seizure clusters and SE are not usually the seizures one wishes to record. They may not be as reliable in determining a patient's usual seizure type, localization, or frequency. Complications of medication withdrawal occasionally include behavioral abnormalities, as well, especially upon carbamazepine withdrawal. [19]

An advantage of inpatient monitoring is the ready availability of clinical staff to assure patient safety, arrange for clinical intervention when necessary, and arrange for additional observation beyond the video. Medications can be administered quickly when necessary, decreasing the risk of anticonvulsant withdrawal-induced seizures or SE. Inpatient monitoring affords readily available EEG technologists to be sure that the recording system is functioning properly throughout the day and to intervene quickly to assure this, e.g., when electrodes become dislodged during epileptic seizures or other events with vigorous movement. Technical problems are frequent and need to be addressed. On-site help can prevent prolonged recordings dominated by artifact. Also, results are usually analyzed more rapidly than with ambulatory monitoring.

Arranging neuroimaging at an ictal or peri-ictal time (such as with ictal SPECT) requires keeping the patient under close observation, usually in a hospital setting. Finally, invasive monitoring cannot be performed on an outpatient basis.

There are also intermediate possibilities. Brief monitoring episodes can be planned in the monitoring unit for patients with frequent daily events, whether seizure, syncope, or other paroxysmal disturbances. Patients whose episodes are precipitated easily by some stimulus may also be suitable for brief monitoring. In general, events occurring less often than daily have a relatively small likelihood of being captured and categorized in a few days' monitoring. Ambulatory recording can be arranged for hospitalized patients who are not necessarily in the epilepsy monitoring unit, e.g., on medical and surgical floors. [20] Monitoring occurs in our clinical research center, connected by cable to the lab, and in the intensive care units to rule out subclinical seizure activity after SE, usually without video.

IV. Practical and Technical Considerations

A baseline EEG should be done before telemetry. It is important to know whether there are background abnormalities or focal or epileptiform features in order to read the studies accurately. This EEG can help sort out the presence or absence of artifacts in the recordings. This is of particular concern when patients are ambulatory and causing movement artifacts that would not normally arise in an EEG laboratory.

Most current ambulatory EEG systems are very similar to those used for inpatient units. Ambulatory monitoring was facilitated markedly by the development of lightweight preamplifiers wrapped near the electrodes on the patient's head that allow amplification without the long wires or cables needed for standard EEGs. [15] These preamplifiers lessen movement artifact. Bipolar recording technique allows for a lower signal amplitude suitable for the preamplifiers.

For seizure onset localization, 16 or more EEG channels are appropriate. Most montages include 18 channels—16 EEG, plus electrocardiogram (ECG), eye movement monitor, or pulse oximeter. Most montages incorporate standard anteroposterior bipolar chains; many use basal electrodes. Montage design depends, in part, on the type of seizure anticipated. One common montage consists of anteroposterior chains; another includes coronal and temporal chains with sphenoidal or additional temporal electrodes incorporated in the coronal chain. When seizures of frontal or generalized origin are suspected, coverage may include more frontal, midline sagittal, and parasagittal leads. Equipment utilizing 32 channels affords greater flexibility in planning which data to acquire.

An important component of most ambulatory EEG systems is a device that allows patients or observers to indicate when symptoms or events are occurring. This can take the form of a pushbutton, which the patient can activate at the onset of typical symptoms. This device is often attached to a waist-worn recorder, which acquires EEG data using a continuous loop design. When the pushbutton is activated, the EEG that was recorded continuously in the prior two minutes is saved (not erased), as is the recording for the next several minutes. Thus, although the system is activated after the onset of symptoms, the EEG can be reviewed from before the time of symptom onset. The description of symptoms can be written on a log sheet for later review.

A portable computer that can perform online analysis is used in ambulatory EEG telemetry for automated detection algorithms. It can be brought home by the patient and kept in close proximity. When the waist-worn recorder is plugged into the computer, data can be analyzed online and the recorder triggered to save EEG segments. For example, each time a suspected electrographic seizure detection occurs, EEG starting two minutes before the detection can be saved; similarly, a brief EEG segment can be saved surrounding each interictal epileptiform discharge (spike or sharp wave) detection.

The portable computer can also be programmed to record routine samples throughout the session to provide a general assessment of EEG background and sleep-wake cycling. When the patient is truly ambulatory and not near the computer, the waist-worn recorder can function independently to record pushbutton activations alone.

Extra basal cranial leads are used often, especially in the search for interictal discharges and seizures of temporal lobe origin. Nasopharyngeal electrodes are too irritating for long-term use. Sphenoidal electrodes are commonly used, particularly when there is concern for a mesial or anterior temporal origin of anticipated seizures. Leaving solid needles in place is not appropriate for long-term monitoring, but flexible stainless steel wires function well and remain safe for up to two weeks. [21] Additional electrode placement, such as in the T1 and T2 positions, can be helpful and appears superior to nasopharyngeal recording.

An ambulatory EEG setup in the EEG laboratory takes about two hours. Electrodes must be attached even more securely to the patient's scalp, with sufficient protection by head wrapping to prevent dislodgement during the more vigorous activities of ambulatory outpatient life. The technologist verifies the integrity of the setup (calibration, electrodes, preamp function, and montage selection) and confirms impedances below 3 kΩ. The baseline recording assures that all components (including event markers and patient-triggered recordings) are functioning properly. The patient is then asked to close her eyes, blink, and so on, to verify electrode position and function. If artifacts occur, the patient can be asked to reproduce the apparent cause by swallowing, chewing, etc. For the monitoring to be useful, sharp features must be clearly differentiable from movement or other artifacts.

Patients and observers are given a detailed equipment instruction guide, a log sheet on which to record the time and description of each event, and 24-hour telephone assistance numbers. Outpatients typically remain on long-term monitoring from one to seven days, with an average of 2.5 days for our lab, whereas inpatients may be monitored for as long as several weeks but average five days. All data are transferred from the home computer and waist-worn recorder into the lab computer daily. Batteries are replaced every 48 hours.

Skilled and experienced EEG technologists are necessary for successful ambulatory event monitoring. Such telemetry requires more technical expertise than routine EEG. In the ambulatory setting and with prolonged recording, problems arise with patients' behavior and equipment function that are generally not seen in routine EEG recording. Intense, time-consuming effort is required to produce reliable and meaningful recordings. Thus, EEG monitoring is more expensive than routine laboratory recording. Still, as noted by Gumnit:

> Even the finest equipment cannot make up for deficiencies in quality of the technical and professional personnel. Unless carried out with consistently high technical standards and provided with interpretations that are clinically reliable. . . . [intensive neurologic monitoring] . . . is simply an expensive waste of time." [2]

Studies should be interpreted by experienced (preferably board-certified) electroencephalographers, and supervision of epilepsy monitoring requires still more intensive training and experience. Reports from monitoring sessions must distinguish clearly what the patient's symptoms were during the events, what was seen by observers and on video monitoring, and what the EEG recording showed at the same time. With the increased potential for artifacts, the variability of clinical seizure manifestations, and the importance of rendering an accurate diagnosis in the case of seizures and in nonepileptic events, a conservative interpretation of results is appropriate.

References

1. Engel J., Burchfiel J., Ebersole J., Gates J., Gotman J., Homan R., Ives J., King D., Lieb J., Sato S., Wilkus R. Long-term monitoring for epilepsy. Report of an IFCN committee. *Electroenceph. Clin. Neurophysiol.* 1993; 87:437–458.

2. Gumnit R. J. Intensive neurodiagnostic monitoring: Summary and recommendations. In: *Advances in Neurology*, Gumnit R. J., ed. New York: Raven Press, 1886; 46:291–302.
3. Mattson R. Intensive neurodiagnostic monitoring: strategy for optimal use. In: *Advances in Neurology*, Gumnit R. J., ed. New York: Raven Press, 1986; 46:281–290.
4. Pierelli, F., Chatrian G. E., Erdly W. W., Swanson P. D. Long-term EEG-video-audio monitoring: detection of partial epileptic seizures and psychogenic episodes by 24-hour EEG record review. *Epilepsia* 1989; 30:513–523.
5. Lesser R. P. Psychogenic seizures. *Neurology* 1996; 46:1499–1507.
6. Reuber M., Pukrop R., Bauer J., Helmstaedter C., Tessendorf N., Elger C. E. Outcome in psychogenic nonepileptic seizures: 1 to 10-year follow-up in 164 patients. *Ann. Neurol.* 2003; 53:305–311.
7. Olson D. M. Success of ambulatory EEG in children. *J. Clin. Neurophysiol.* 2001; 18:158–161.
8. Ebersole J. S., Leroy R. F. Evaluation of ambulatory cassette EEG monitoring: III. Diagnostic accuracy compared to intensive inpatient EEG monitoring. *Neurology* 1983; 33:853–860.
9. Schomer D. L., Ives J. R., Schachter S. C. The role of ambulatory EEG in the evaluation of patients for epilepsy surgery. *J. Clin. Neurophysiol.* 1999; 16:116–129.
10. DeLorenzo R. J., Waterhouse E. J., Towne A. R., Boggs J. G., Ko D., DeLorenzo G. A., Brown A., Garnett L. Persistent nonconvulsive status epilepticus after the control of convulsive status epilepticus. *Epilepsia* 1998; 39:833–840.
11. Towne A. R., Pellock J. M., Ko D., DeLorenzo, R. J. Determinants of mortality in status epilepticus. *Epilepsia* 1994; 35:27–34.
12. Drislane F. W., Schomer D. L. Clinical implications of generalized electrographic status epilepticus. *Epilepsy Res.* 1994; 19:111–121.
13. So E. L., Ruggles K. H., Ahmann P. A., Trudeau S. K., Weatherford K. J., Trenerry M. R. Clinical significance and outcome of subclinical status epilepticus in adults. *J. Epilepsy* 1995; 8:11–15.
14. Bazil C. W., Kothari M., Luciano D., Moroney J., Song S., Vasquez B., Weinreb H. J., Devinsky O. Provocation of nonepileptic seizures by suggestion in a general seizure population. *Epilepsia* 1994; 35:768–770.
15. Ives J. R., Thompson C. J., Gloor P. Seizure monitoring: a new tool in electroencephalography. *Electroenceph. Clin. Neurophysiol.* 1976; 41:422–427.
16. Riley T. L., Porter R. J., White B. G., Penry J. K. The hospital experience and seizure control. *Neurology* 1981; 31:912–915.
17. Chang B. S., Ives J. R., Schomer D. L., Drislane F. W. Outpatient EEG monitoring in the presurgical evaluation of patients with refractory temporal lobe epilepsy. *J. Clin. Neurophysiol.* 2002; 19:152–156.
18. Rose A. B., McCabe P. H., Gilliam F. G., Smith B. J., Boggs J. G., Ficker D. M., Moore J. L., Passaro E. A., Bazil C. W. Occurrence of seizure clusters and status epilepticus during inpatient video-EEG monitoring. *Neurology* 2003; 60:975–978.
19. Malow B. A., Blaxton T. A., Shertz B., Theodore W. H. Carbamazepine withdrawal: Effects of taper rate on seizure frequency. *Neurology* 1993; 43:2280–2284.
20. Shihabuddin B., Abou-Khalil B., Fakhoury T. The value of combined ambulatory cassette-EEG and video monitoring in the differential diagnosis of intractable seizures. *Clin. Neurophysiol.* 1999; 110:1452–1457.
21. Ives J. R., Gloor P. Update: chronic sphenoidal electrodes. *Electroenceph. Clin. Neurophysiol.* 1978; 44:789–790.

TECHNICAL ASPECTS

TECHNICAL 1

A Typical Screen or Printed Page of Ambulatory EEG Recording

This page demonstrates the typical set of labels, annotations, and data that accompany a single screen or printed page of ambulatory EEG recording. Specifics vary depending on the recording equipment vendor and display software.

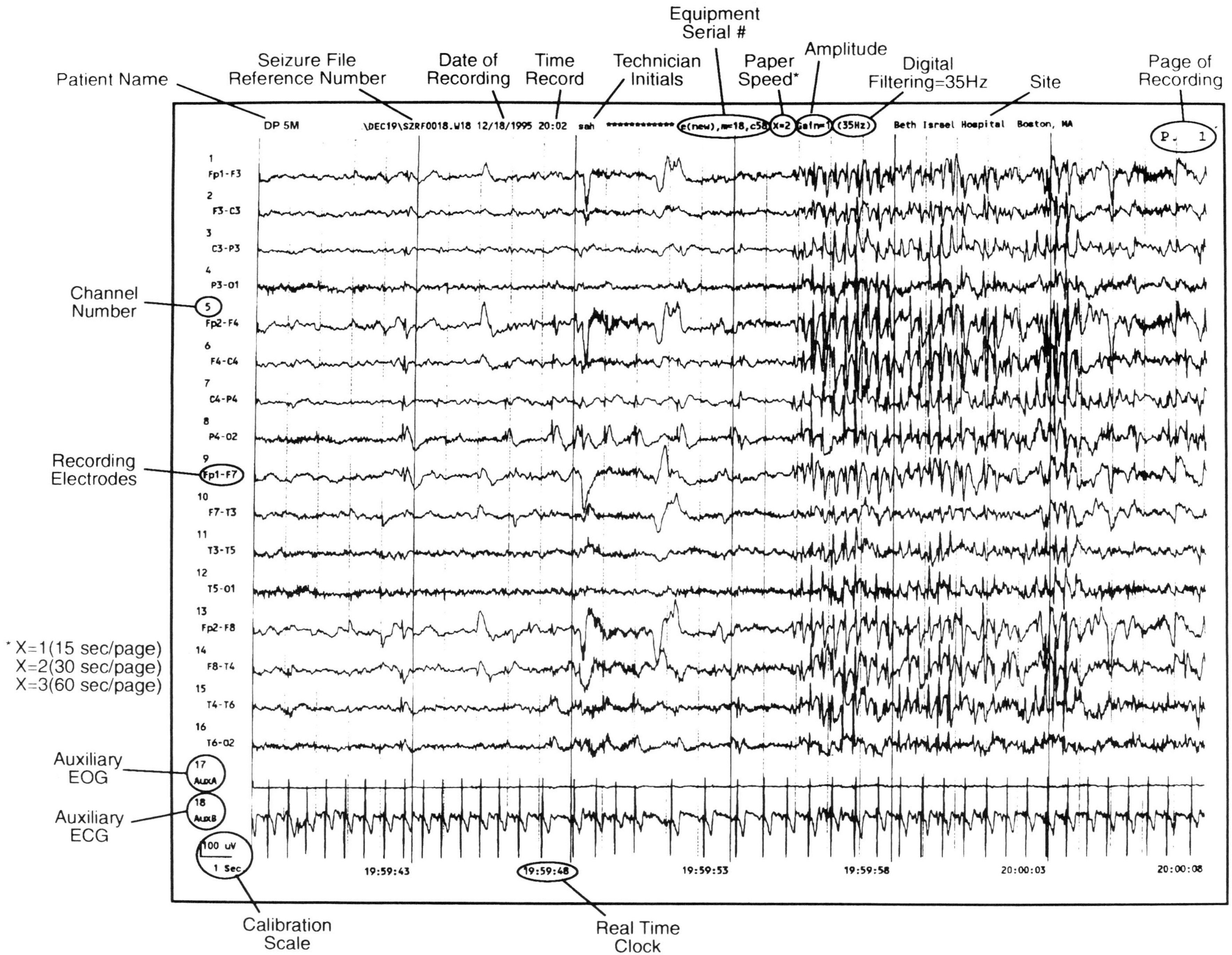

Equipment Serial #
Amplitude
Patient Name
Seizure File Reference Number
Date of Recording
Time Record
Technician Initials
Paper Speed*
Digital Filtering=35Hz
Site
Page of Recording
DP 5M
\DEC19\SZRF0018.W18 12/18/1995 20:02 sah
e(new),m=18,c5
X=2
Gain=1
(35Hz)
Beth Israel Hospital Boston, MA
P. 1
Channel Number
Recording Electrodes
1 Fp1-F3
2 F3-C3
3 C3-P3
4 P3-O1
5 Fp2-F4
6 F4-C4
7 C4-P4
8 P4-O2
9 Fp1-F7
10 F7-T3
11 T3-T5
12 T5-O1
13 Fp2-F8
14 F8-T4
15 T4-T6
16 T6-O2
17 AUXA
18 AUXB
* X=1(15 sec/page)
X=2(30 sec/page)
X=3(60 sec/page)
Auxiliary EOG
Auxiliary ECG
100 uV
1 Sec
19:59:43
19:59:48
19:59:53
19:59:58
20:00:03
20:00:08
Calibration Scale
Real Time Clock

Left Temporal Seizure: No Filter Used

This excerpt, which represents the beginning of a left temporally predominant seizure, is shown with no filtering. The upper bandwidth of this system is approximately 100 Hz based on the 200-Hz sampling frequency of the data acquisition.

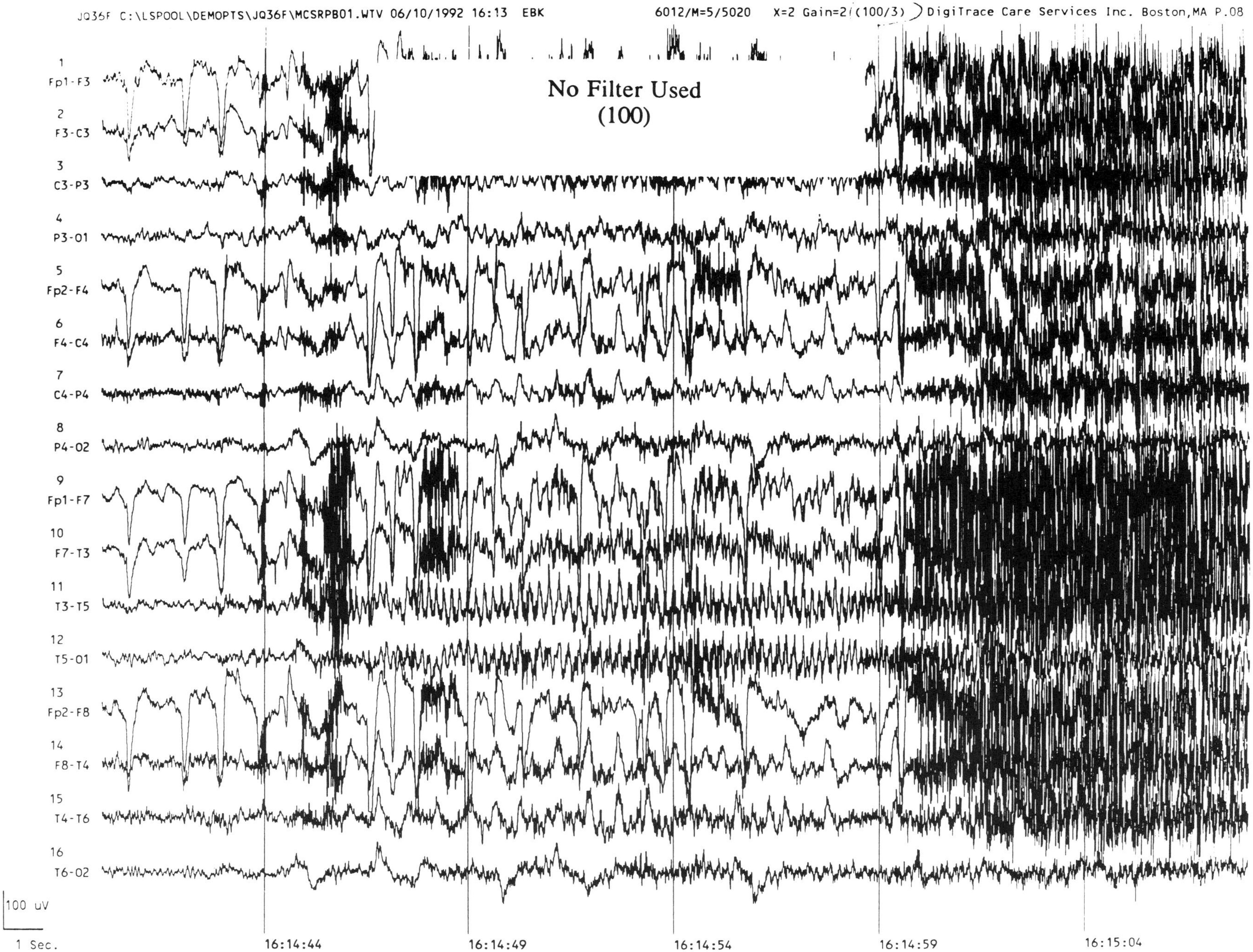
JQ36F C:\LSPOOL\DEMOPTS\JQ36F\MCSRPB01.WTV 06/10/1992 16:13 EBK
6012/M=5/5020 X=2 Gain=2 (100/3) DigiTrace Care Services Inc. Boston,MA P.08
No Filter Used
(100)
1 Fp1-F3
2 F3-C3
3 C3-P3
4 P3-O1
5 Fp2-F4
6 F4-C4
7 C4-P4
8 P4-O2
9 Fp1-F7
10 F7-T3
11 T3-T5
12 T5-O1
13 Fp2-F8
14 F8-T4
15 T4-T6
16 T6-O2
100 uV
1 Sec.
16:14:44
16:14:49
16:14:54
16:14:59
16:15:04

TECHNICAL 3

Left Temporal Seizure: 60-Hz Notch Filter

This excerpt represents the same recording as in the prior figure, now displayed with a "double" notched 60-Hz filter. Electrical activity near the 60-Hz frequency has been extracted but activity above and below 60-Hz is unaffected. Comparison to the prior figure reveals that the 60-Hz filter has extracted a moderate amount of fast activity.

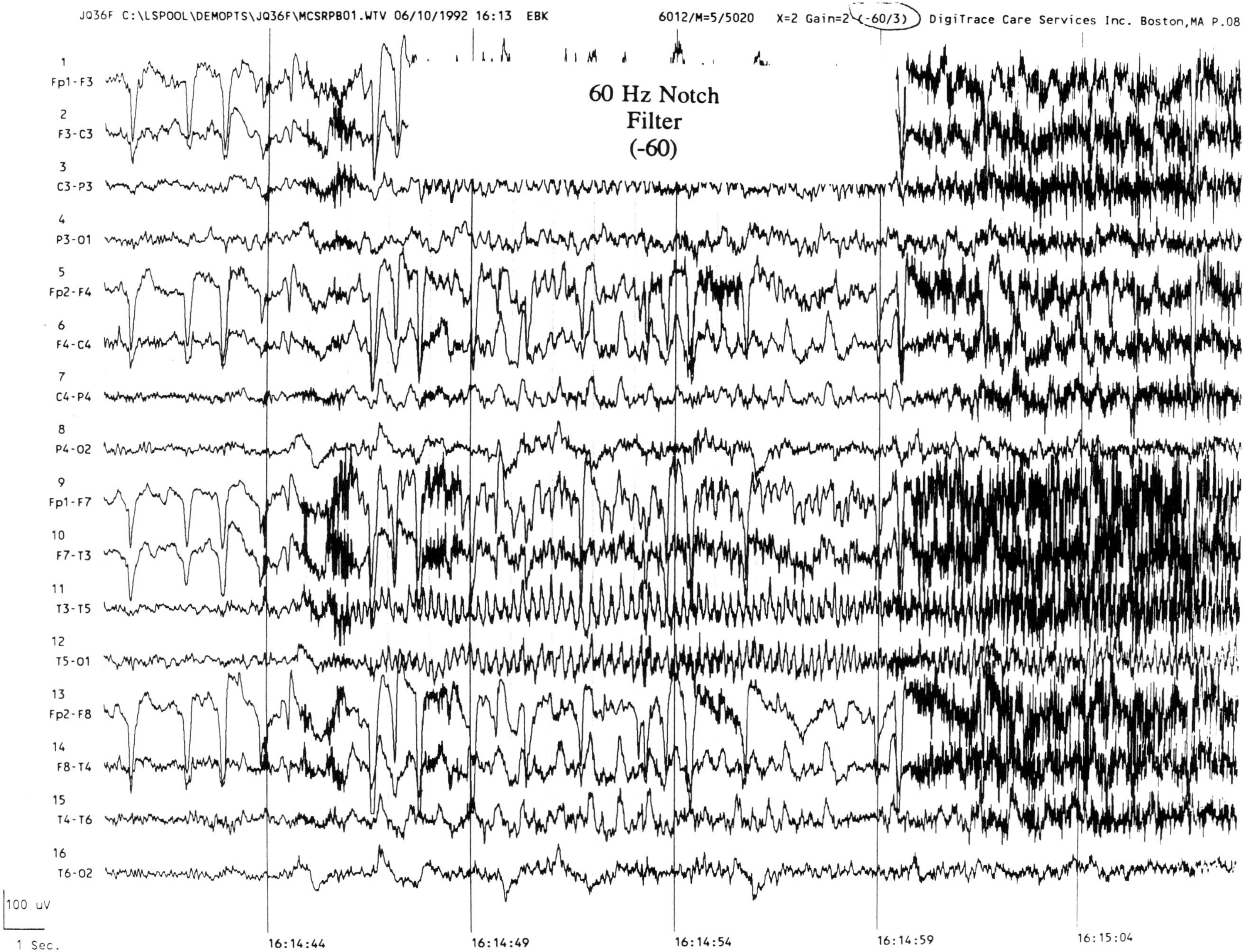
JQ36F C:\LSPOOL\DEMOPTS\JQ36F\MCSRPB01.WTV 06/10/1992 16:13 EBK
6012/M=5/5020 X=2 Gain=2 (-60/3) DigiTrace Care Services Inc. Boston,MA P.08
60 Hz Notch Filter (-60)
1 Fp1-F3
2 F3-C3
3 C3-P3
4 P3-O1
5 Fp2-F4
6 F4-C4
7 C4-P4
8 P4-O2
9 Fp1-F7
10 F7-T3
11 T3-T5
12 T5-O1
13 Fp2-F8
14 F8-T4
15 T4-T6
16 T6-O2
100 uV
1 Sec.
16:14:44
16:14:49
16:14:54
16:14:59
16:15:04

Left Temporal Seizure: High Frequency 35-Hz Filter

This excerpt represents the same recording as in the prior figure, now displayed with the high frequency filter setting set at 35 Hz. Comparison to the prior figure reveals that this figure appears to have removed a considerable amount of the fast activity seen during the last 10 seconds of this record, without altering the appearance of the earlier slower frequency activity.

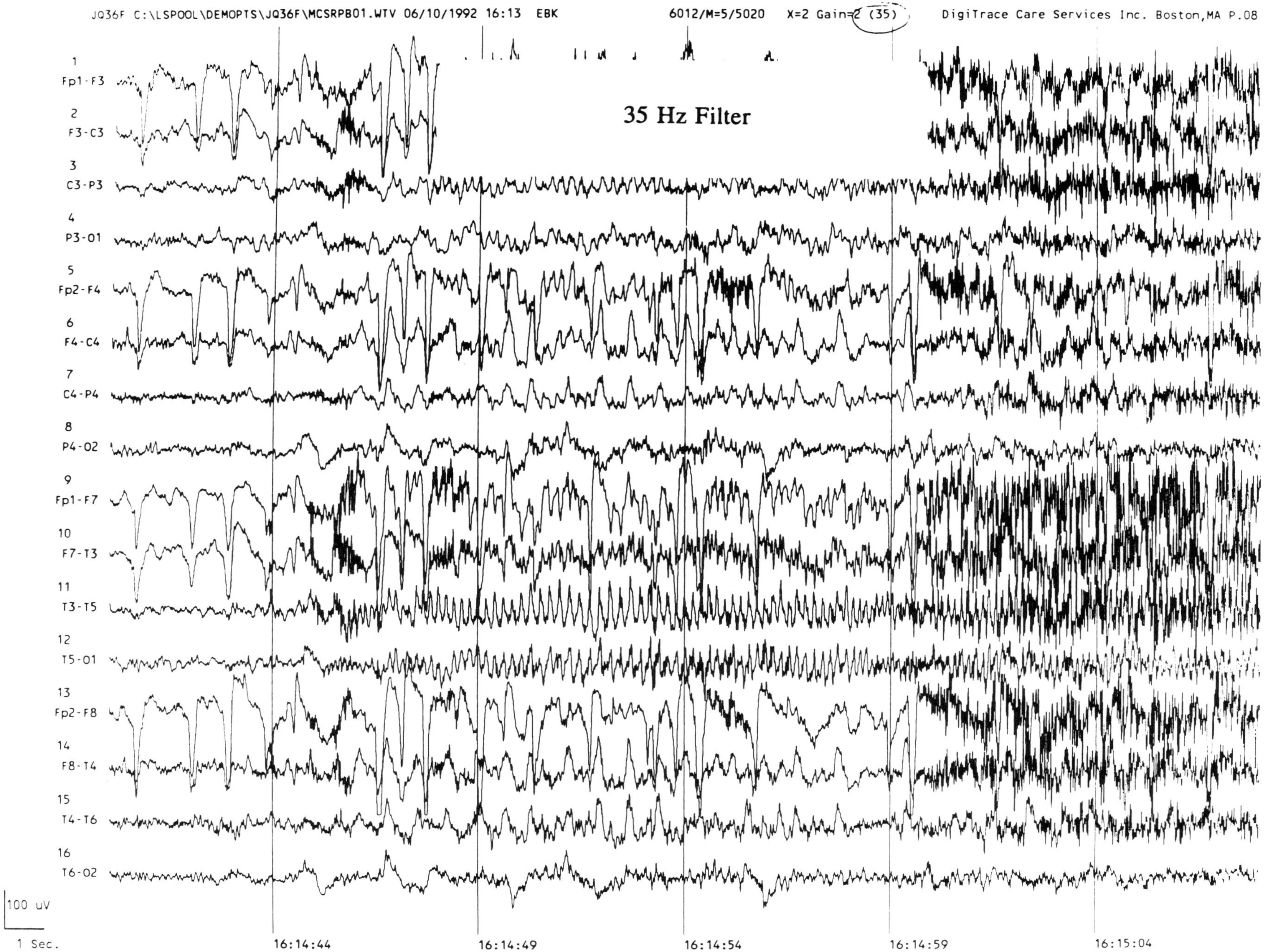
JQ36F C:\LSPOOL\DEMOPTS\JQ36F\MCSRPB01.WTV 06/10/1992 16:13 EBK
6012/M=5/5020 X=2 Gain=2 (35)
DigiTrace Care Services Inc. Boston,MA P.08
35 Hz Filter
1 Fp1-F3
2 F3-C3
3 C3-P3
4 P3-O1
5 Fp2-F4
6 F4-C4
7 C4-P4
8 P4-O2
9 Fp1-F7
10 F7-T3
11 T3-T5
12 T5-O1
13 Fp2-F8
14 F8-T4
15 T4-T6
16 T6-O2
100 uV
1 Sec.
16:14:44
16:14:49
16:14:54
16:14:59
16:15:04

TECHNICAL 5

Left Temporal Seizure: High Frequency 15-Hz Filter

This excerpt represents the same recording as in the prior figure, now displayed with a high-frequency filter set at 15 Hz. This further filtering of higher frequency activity improves the "readability" of the record. Electroencephalographers reviewing ambulatory EEG monitoring may find it helpful to review ictal recordings with different filter settings to look for different frequency-related activity, as long as the inherent limitations of filtering are recognized.

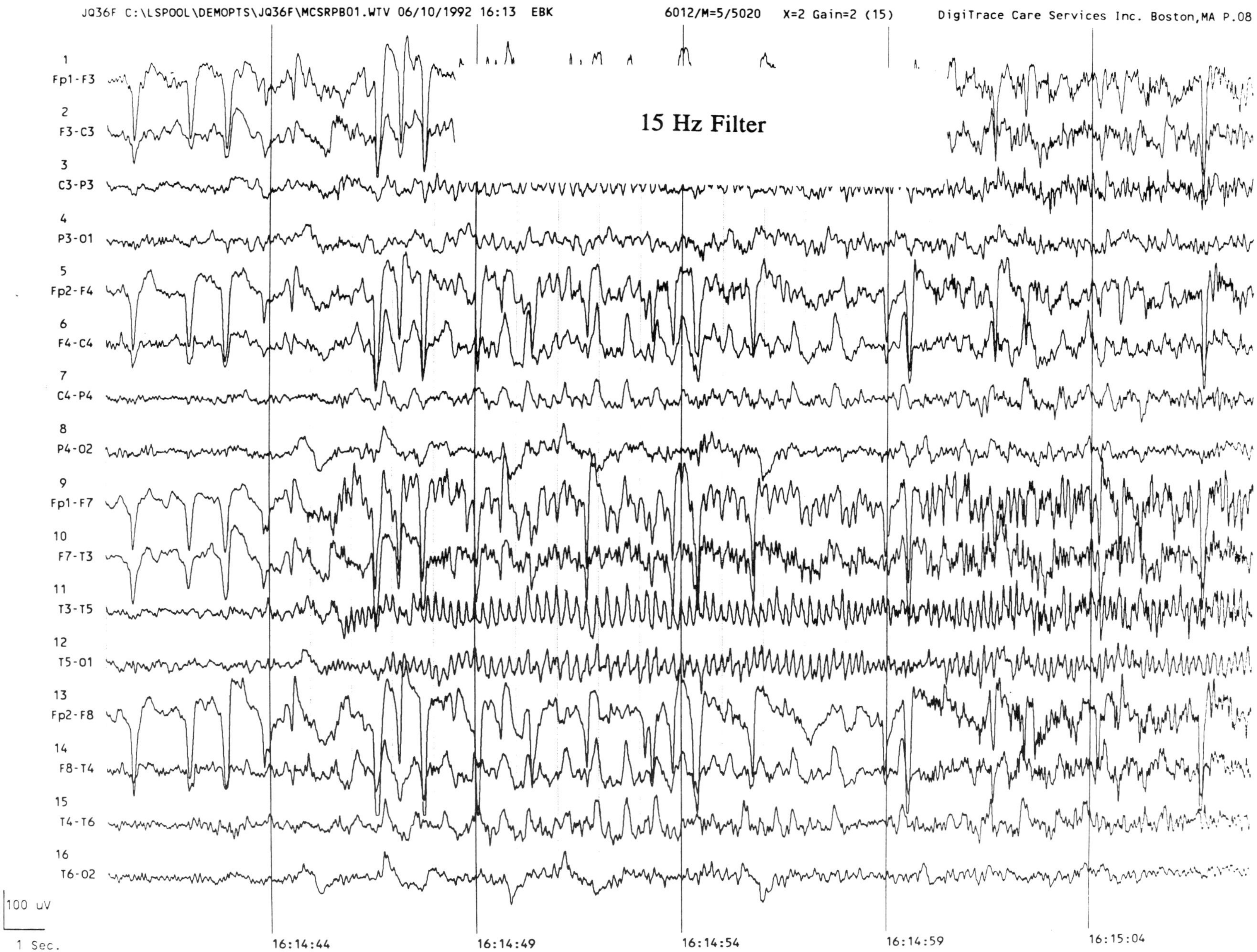
JQ36F C:\LSPOOL\DEMOPTS\JQ36F\MCSRPB01.WTV 06/10/1992 16:13 EBK
6012/M=5/5020 X=2 Gain=2 (15)
DigiTrace Care Services Inc. Boston,MA P.08
15 Hz Filter
1 Fp1-F3
2 F3-C3
3 C3-P3
4 P3-O1
5 Fp2-F4
6 F4-C4
7 C4-P4
8 P4-O2
9 Fp1-F7
10 F7-T3
11 T3-T5
12 T5-O1
13 Fp2-F8
14 F8-T4
15 T4-T6
16 T6-O2
100 uV
1 Sec.
16:14:44
16:14:49
16:14:54
16:14:59
16:15:04

TECHNICAL 6

Generalized Spike-Wave Activity: Paper Speed 30 Seconds Per Page

This excerpt represents a burst of generalized 3-per-second spike-and-wave activity displayed at a paper speed of 30 seconds per page. The vertical lines are spaced 5 seconds apart.

CH9F C:\CH9F\SZRF0012.WTV 01/30/1992 21:40 KKB ************ E=02,18=25,c=28 X=2 Gain=1 (100/3) DigiTrace Care Services Inc. Boston,MA P.01

File Printed
with Paper Speed
at 30 Seconds/Page

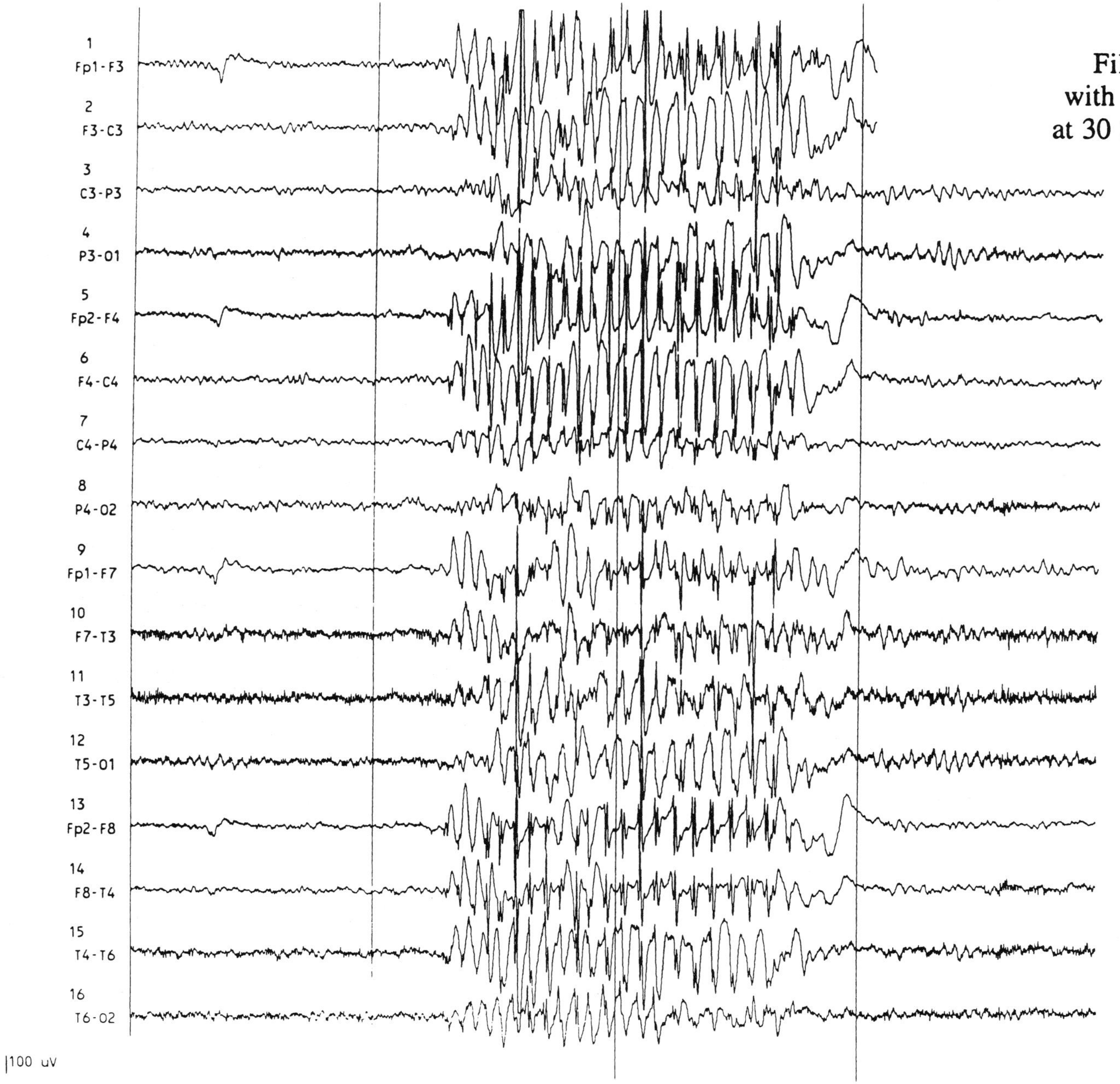

Generalized Spike-Wave Activity: Paper Speed 15 Seconds Per Page

This excerpt represents the same recording as in the prior figure, now displayed with a paper speed of 15 seconds per page. The vertical lines are spaced 5 seconds apart.

CH9F C:\CH9F\SZRF0012.WTV 01/30/1992 21:40 KKB ************ E=02,18=25,c=28 X=1 Gain=1 (100/3) DigiTrace Care Services Inc. Boston,MA P.01

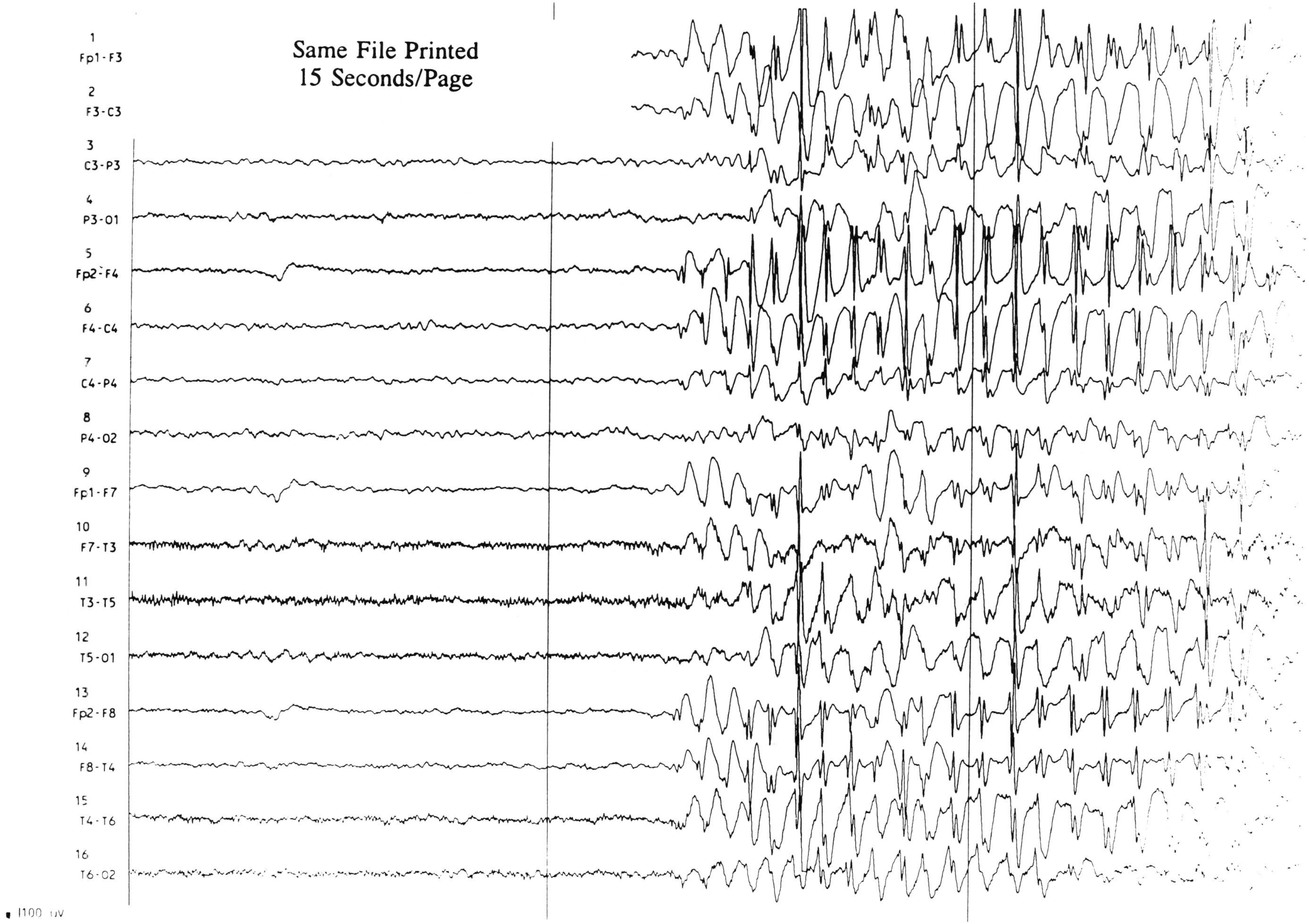

Generalized Spike-Wave Activity: Gain = 2

This excerpt represents the same recording as in the prior figure, now displayed with a gain of 2. The scale in the lower left corner indicates the height of 100 microvolt activity.

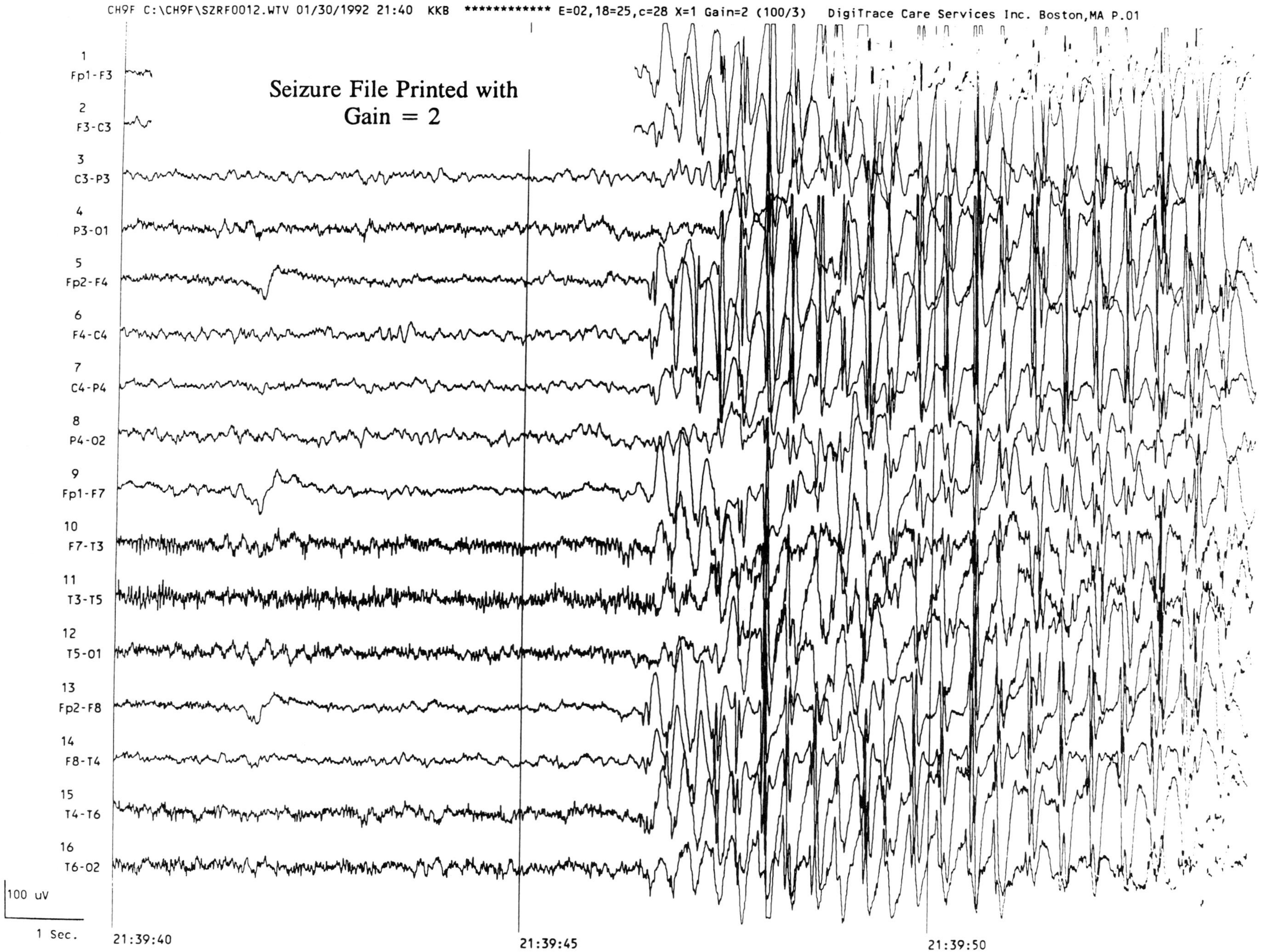
CH9F C:\CH9F\SZRF0012.WTV 01/30/1992 21:40 KKB ************ E=02,18=25,c=28 X=1 Gain=2 (100/3) DigiTrace Care Services Inc. Boston,MA P.01
Seizure File Printed with
Gain = 2
1 Fp1-F3
2 F3-C3
3 C3-P3
4 P3-O1
5 Fp2-F4
6 F4-C4
7 C4-P4
8 P4-O2
9 Fp1-F7
10 F7-T3
11 T3-T5
12 T5-O1
13 Fp2-F8
14 F8-T4
15 T4-T6
16 T6-O2
100 uV
1 Sec.
21:39:40
21:39:45
21:39:50

Generalized Spike-Wave Activity: Gain = 1

This excerpt represents the same recording as in the prior figure, now displayed with a gain of 1. Comparison to the prior figure reveals that the height of 100 microvolt activity is half that seen in the prior figure, according to the scale in the lower left corner.

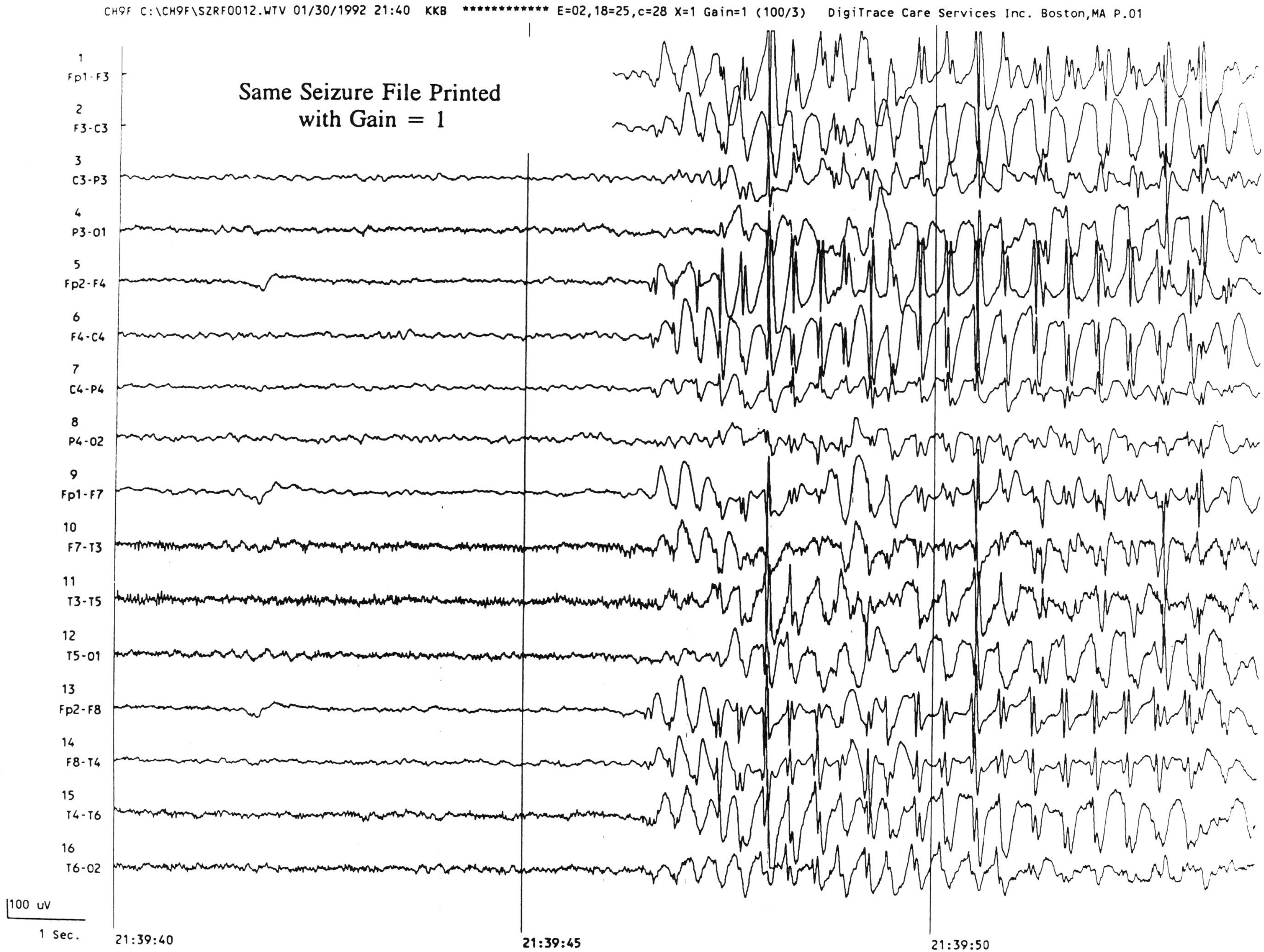
CH9F C:\CH9F\SZRF0012.WTV 01/30/1992 21:40 KKB ************ E=02,18=25,c=28 X=1 Gain=1 (100/3) DigiTrace Care Services Inc. Boston,MA P.01
Same Seizure File Printed
with Gain = 1
1 Fp1-F3
2 F3-C3
3 C3-P3
4 P3-O1
5 Fp2-F4
6 F4-C4
7 C4-P4
8 P4-O2
9 Fp1-F7
10 F7-T3
11 T3-T5
12 T5-O1
13 Fp2-F8
14 F8-T4
15 T4-T6
16 T6-O2
100 uV
1 Sec.
21:39:40
21:39:45
21:39:50

NORMAL SLEEP MORPHOLOGIES

Sleep Spindles

The electroencephalographer reviewing ambulatory EEG recordings must become familiar with standard sleep morphologies and their appearance on ambulatory EEG. In this excerpt, a symmetric sleep spindle is seen at 22:02:54.

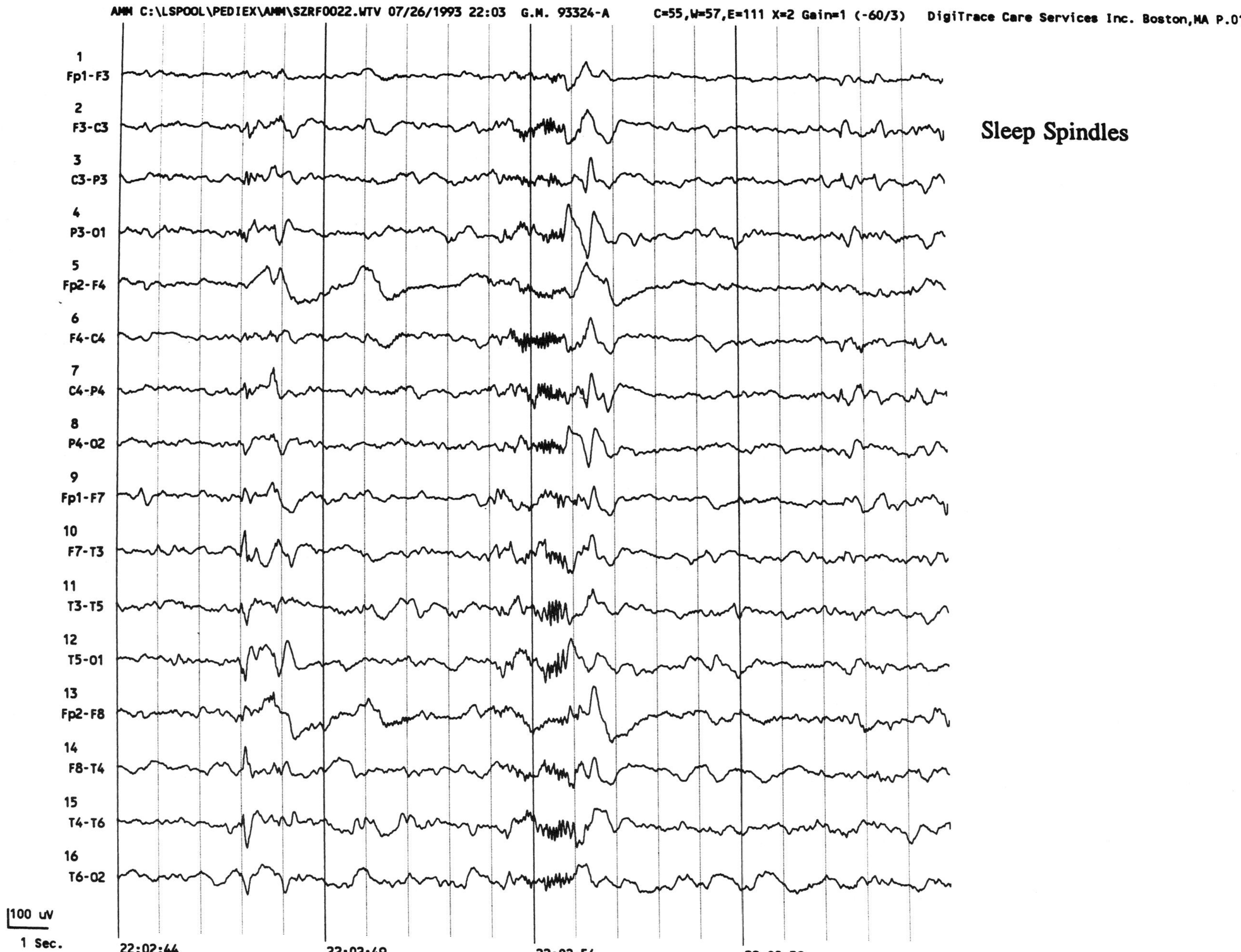

Sleep Spindles

K-Complexes and Sleep Spindles Recorded by Spike Detection Algorithm

Spike detection algorithms, which are often programmed to capture files during the nighttime hours, can be triggered by normal sleep morphologies, including the K-complexes and sleep spindles seen here.

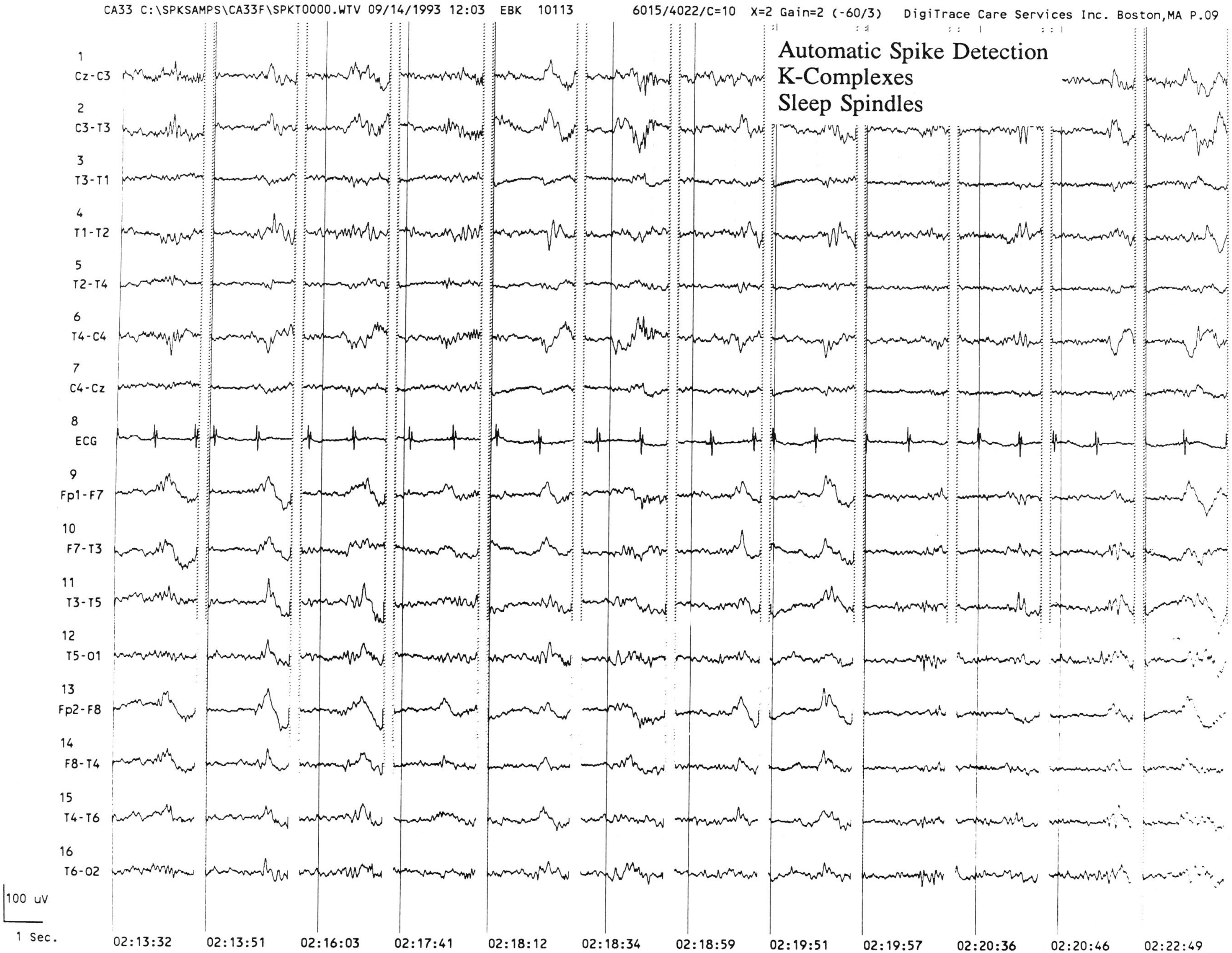
CA33 C:\SPKSAMPS\CA33F\SPKT0000.WTV 09/14/1993 12:03 EBK 10113
6015/4022/C=10 X=2 Gain=2 (-60/3)
DigiTrace Care Services Inc. Boston,MA P.09
Automatic Spike Detection
K-Complexes
Sleep Spindles
1 Cz-C3
2 C3-T3
3 T3-T1
4 T1-T2
5 T2-T4
6 T4-C4
7 C4-Cz
8 ECG
9 Fp1-F7
10 F7-T3
11 T3-T5
12 T5-O1
13 Fp2-F8
14 F8-T4
15 T4-T6
16 T6-O2
100 uV
1 Sec.
02:13:32
02:13:51
02:16:03
02:17:41
02:18:12
02:18:34
02:18:59
02:19:51
02:19:57
02:20:36
02:20:46
02:22:49

Rapid Eye Movement of Sleep

Rapid eye movements during sleep, such as the horizontal movements seen at 18:48:23 and 18:48:30 in this excerpt, can lead to artifact on ambulatory EEG recordings that might mimic frontal or anterior temporal cerebral potentials.

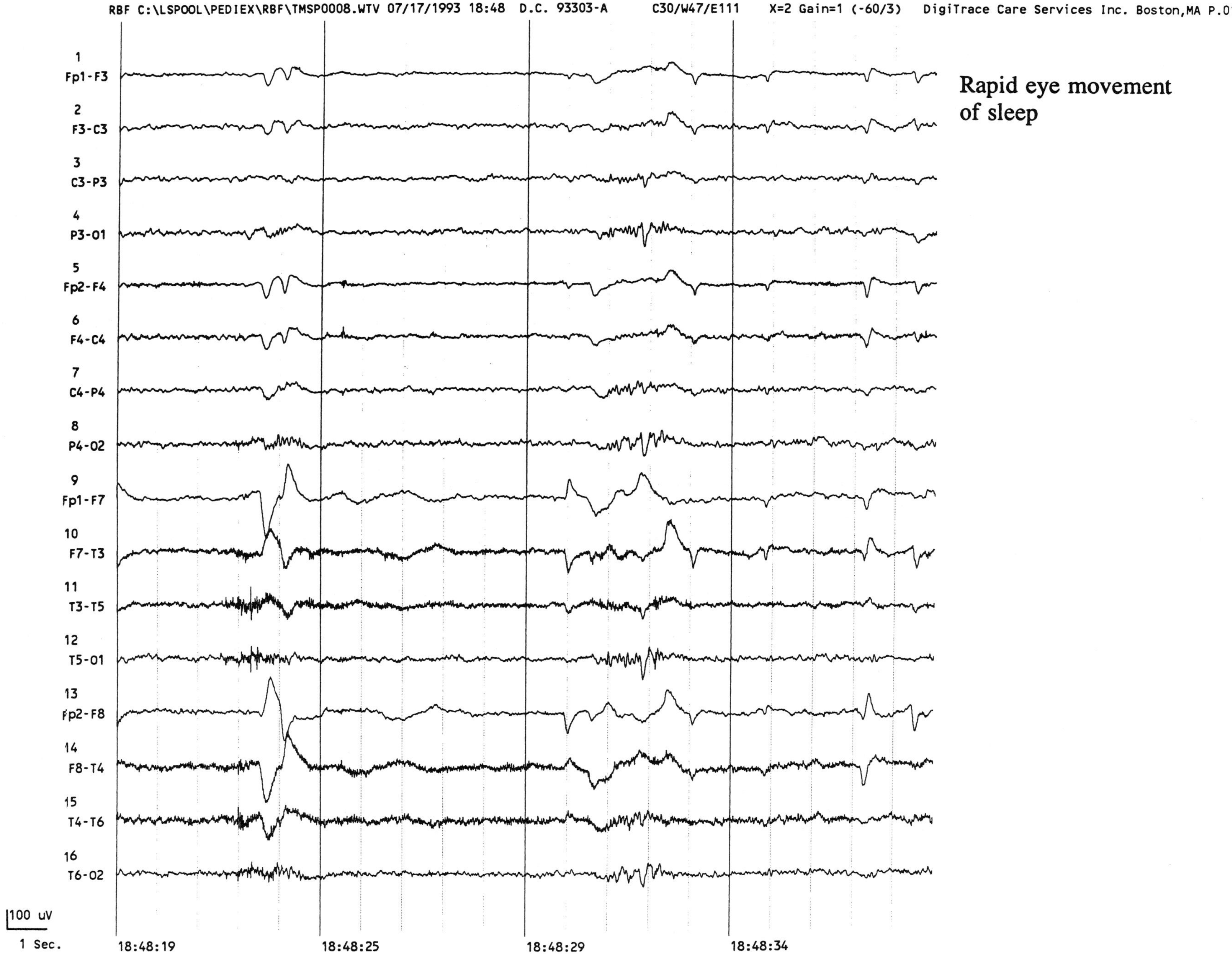

Rapid eye movement of sleep

AMBULATORY ARTIFACTS

Horizontal Eye Movement and Blink Artifacts

Two types of eye movement artifact are seen. Channel 8 is designated as an eye monitor channel and records from electrodes placed over the right and left lateral epicanthal sites. A horizontal eye movement at about 16:49:56 is seen in both channel 4 (T1–T2) and in channel 8 (eye monitor). Blink artifacts, noted repeatedly from 16:49:57 to 16:50:04, are well-seen in the frontal channels but not in channel 8.

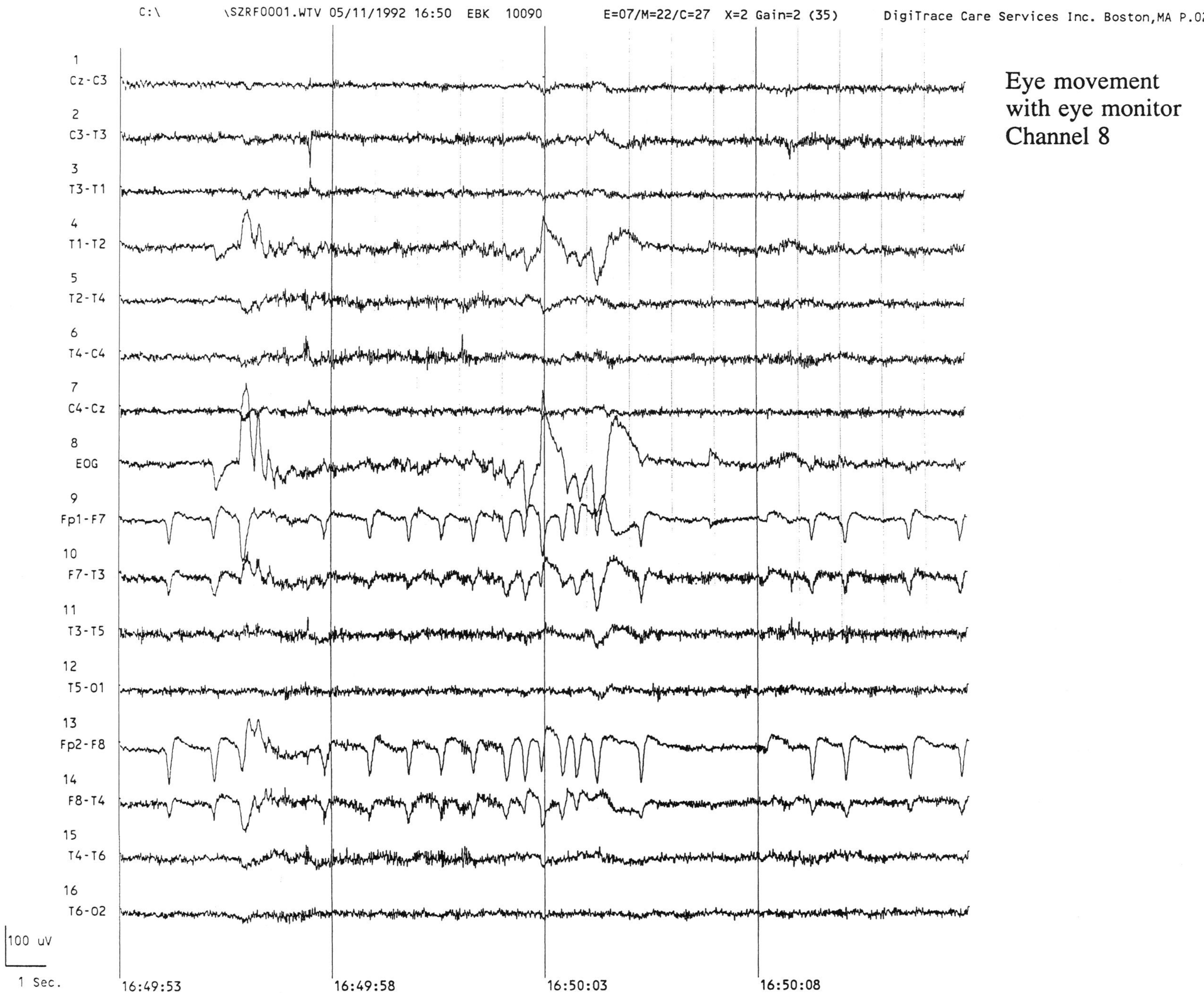

Eye movement with eye monitor Channel 8

Eye-Blink Artifact

Repetitive eye blinking is seen best in the frontal channels throughout this excerpt.

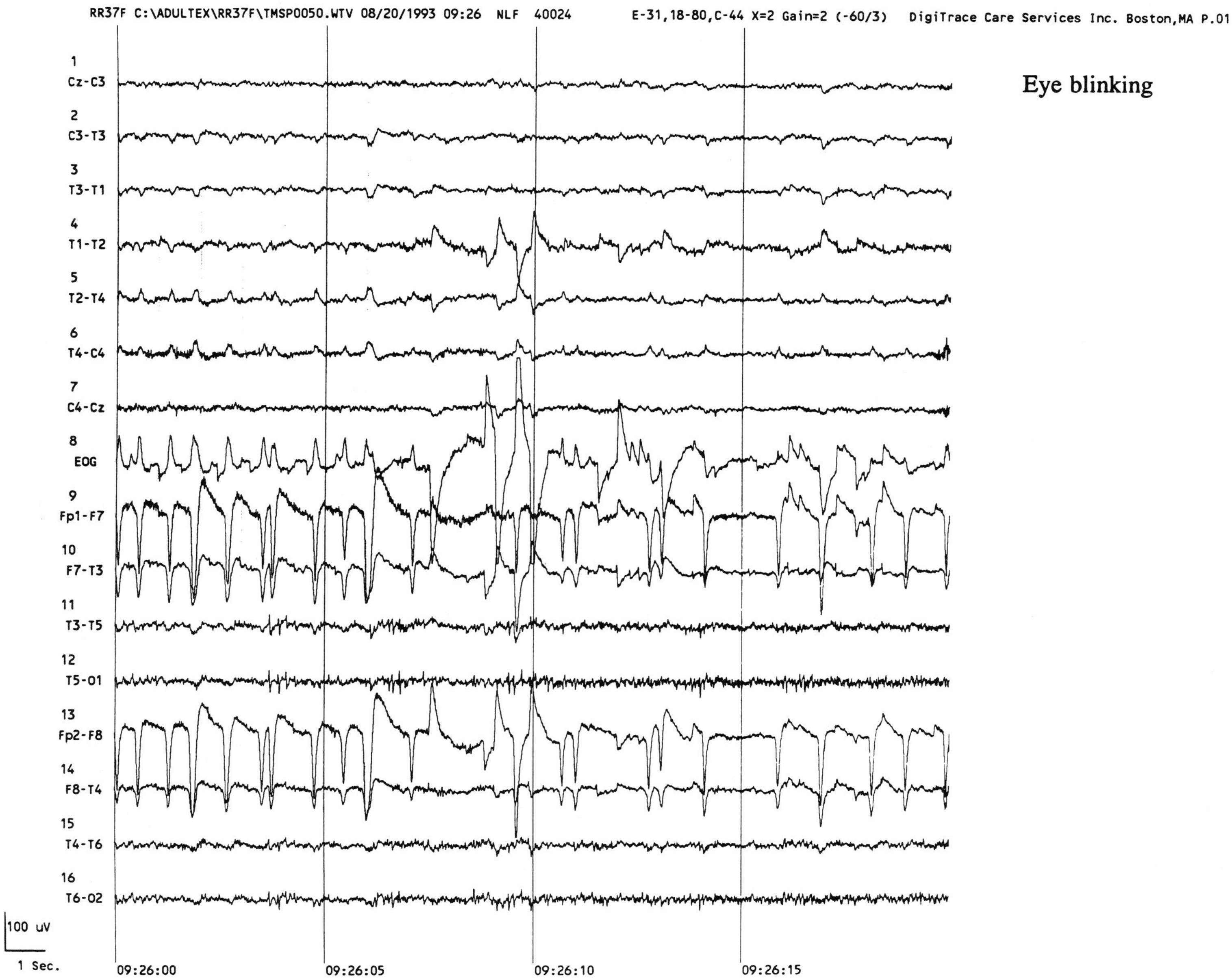

Eye blinking

Eye Flutter Artifact Recorded by Seizure Detection Algorithm

Rhythmic eye flutter can occur at quite high frequencies, in this case 5–8 Hz, and trigger automated seizure detection algorithms. Here, the algorithm captured an episode of eye flutter beginning at 19:27:02. In the absence of video, eye flutter artifact can be distinguished from ictal events in a number of electrographic ways, including the lack of evolution in frequency or amplitude over time.

MM34 C:\SP_SAMPS\MM34\SZRF0001.WTV 10/08/1991 19:28 EBK 10012 ? Seizures X=2 Gain=2 (-60/3) DigiTrace Care Services Inc. Boston,MA P.01

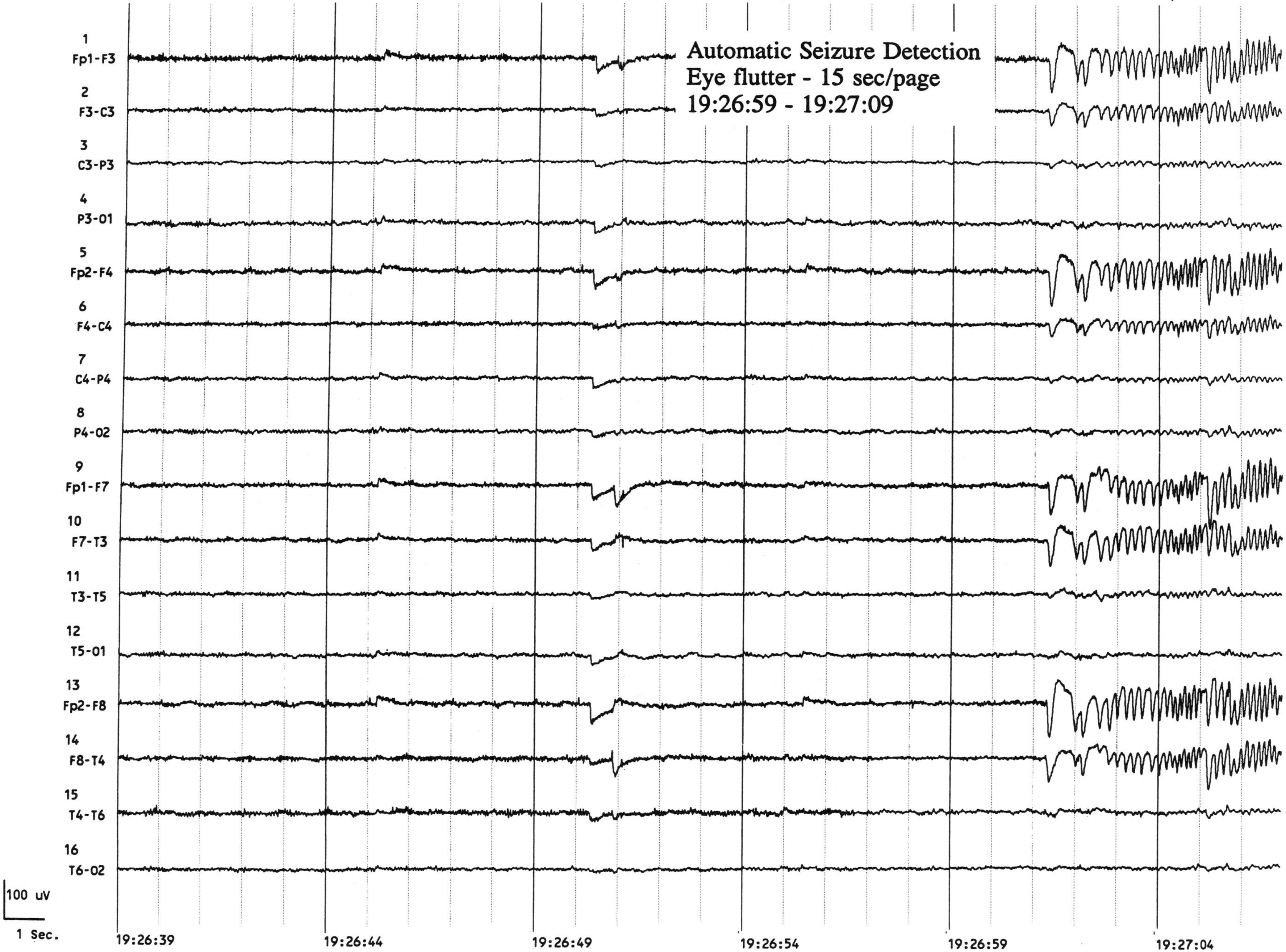

Electrode Tapping Artifact

With ambulatory EEG recording, there may be periods in which the patient is scratching or pressing on the scalp electrodes. Concomitant video recording would clearly demonstrate this, but in the absence of video, the electroencephalographer must be alert to the possibility of this kind of artifact. Here, the O2 electrode is being tapped or scratched by the patient from about 22:11:05 to 22:11:11. Only the channel including O2 is affected and there is no electrical field to this artifact.

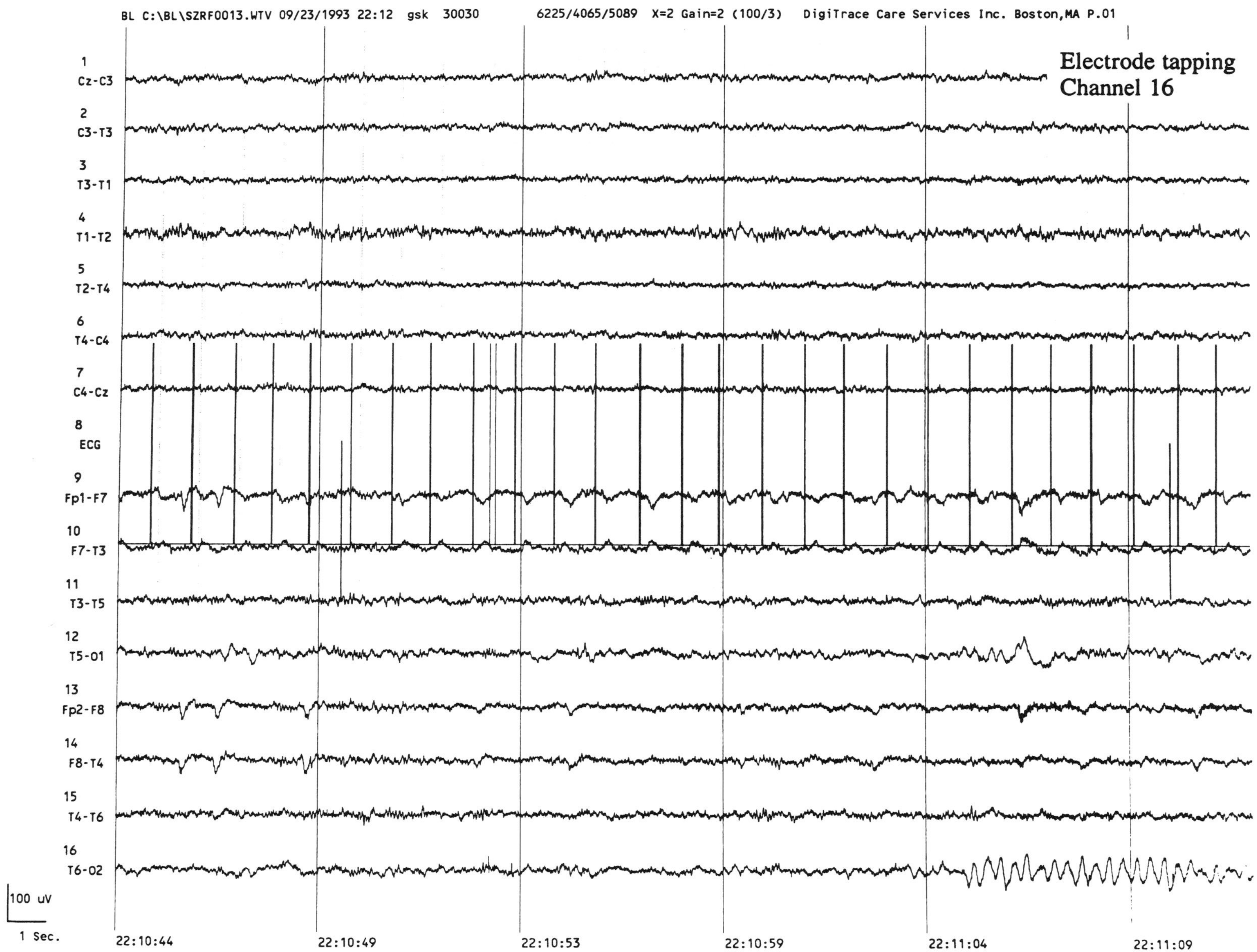
BL C:\BL\SZRF0013.WTV 09/23/1993 22:12 gsk 30030 6225/4065/5089 X=2 Gain=2 (100/3) DigiTrace Care Services Inc. Boston,MA P.01
Electrode tapping
Channel 16
1 Cz-C3
2 C3-T3
3 T3-T1
4 T1-T2
5 T2-T4
6 T4-C4
7 C4-Cz
8 ECG
9 Fp1-F7
10 F7-T3
11 T3-T5
12 T5-O1
13 Fp2-F8
14 F8-T4
15 T4-T6
16 T6-O2
100 uV
1 Sec.
22:10:44
22:10:49
22:10:53
22:10:59
22:11:04
22:11:09

Jaw-Clenching Artifact

Periods of jaw clenching and biting during ambulatory EEG recording can be associated with artifact. This activity is often most prominent over the temporal regions, presumably due to temporalis or masseter muscle contraction. In the absence of video recording, it is useful to ask patients to refrain from chewing gum and to record the timing of meals. Here, such artifact is seen from 11:44:10 through the end of the excerpt and appears most prominently over the right temporal region.

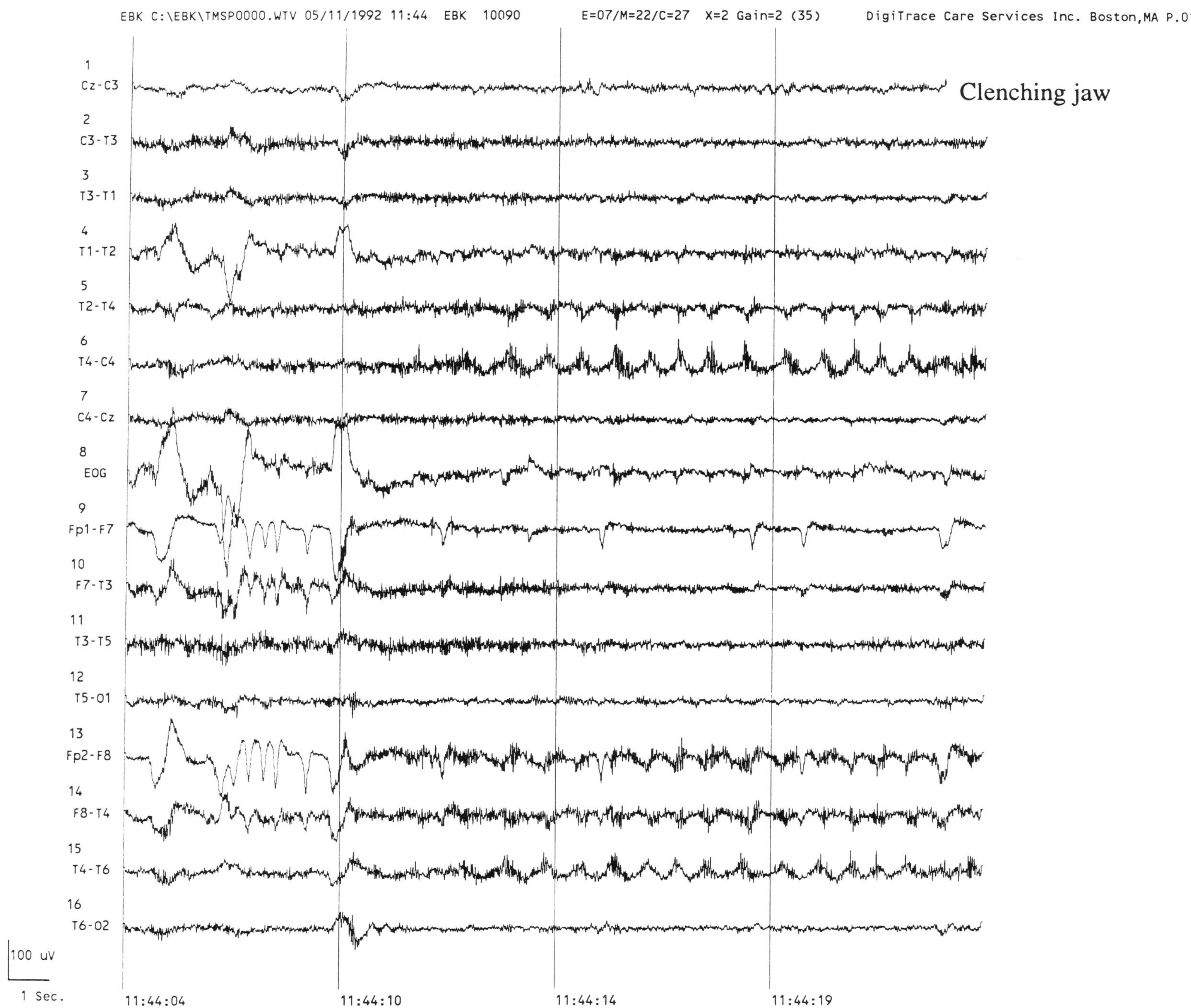

Clenching jaw

Chewing Artifact

Chewing artifact can often have rhythmic features and at times may resemble ictal activity. Here, artifact begins at 21:59:35 and is characterized by the rhythmic appearance of muscle artifact centered mostly over the temporal regions bilaterally.

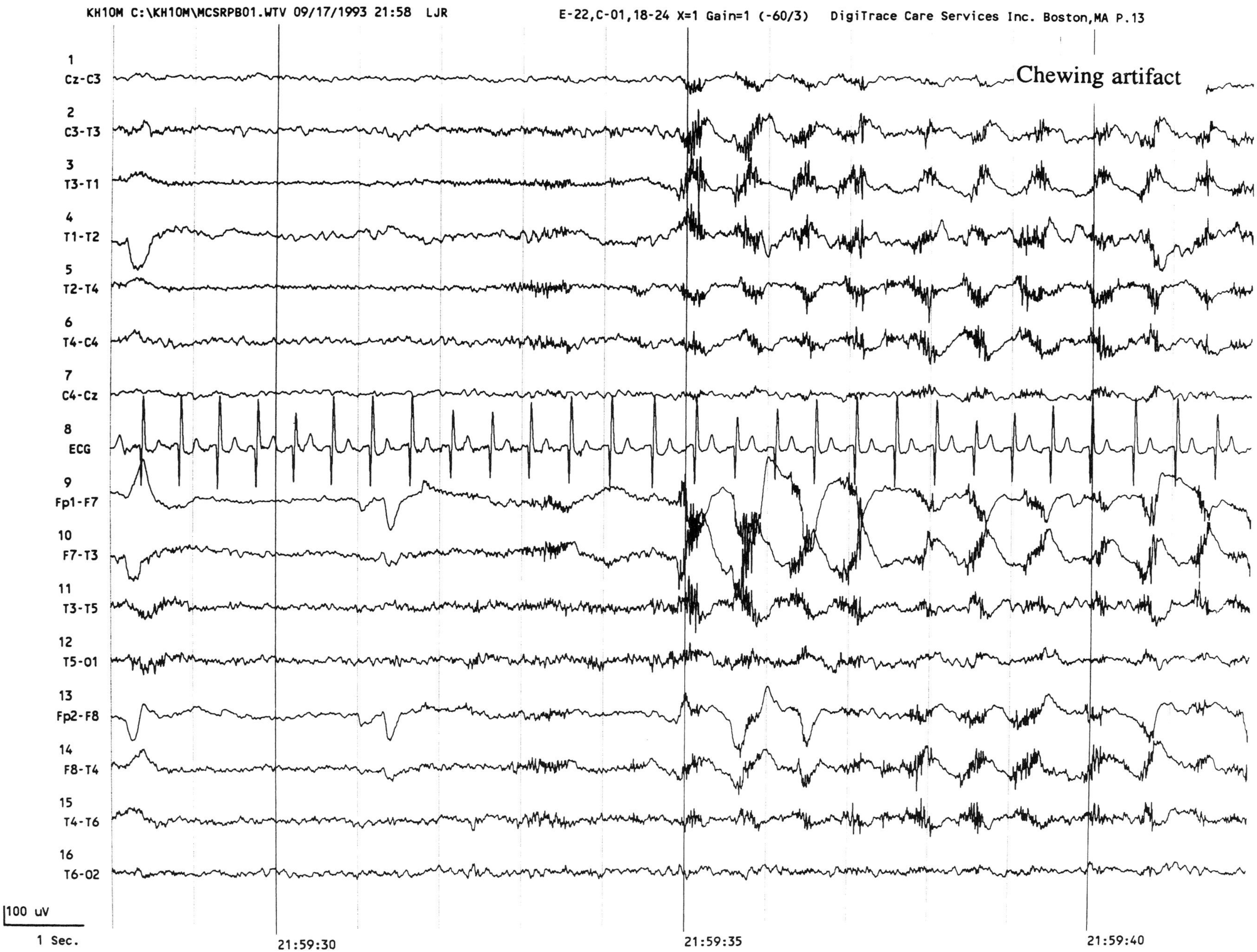
KH10M C:\KH10M\MCSRPB01.WTV 09/17/1993 21:58 LJR
E-22,C-01,18-24 X=1 Gain=1 (-60/3)
DigiTrace Care Services Inc. Boston,MA P.13
Chewing artifact
1 Cz-C3
2 C3-T3
3 T3-T1
4 T1-T2
5 T2-T4
6 T4-C4
7 C4-Cz
8 ECG
9 Fp1-F7
10 F7-T3
11 T3-T5
12 T5-O1
13 Fp2-F8
14 F8-T4
15 T4-T6
16 T6-O2
100 uV
1 Sec.
21:59:30
21:59:35
21:59:40

Chewing Artifact Recorded by Spike Detection Algorithm

Chewing artifact can have rhythmic and sharp features, and can thus be picked up by automated detection algorithms (see Chapter 2). Here, the spike detections at 23:53:23 and at 23:53:34 capture high-frequency sharp waveforms that are artifactual in nature, in association with a nighttime snack.

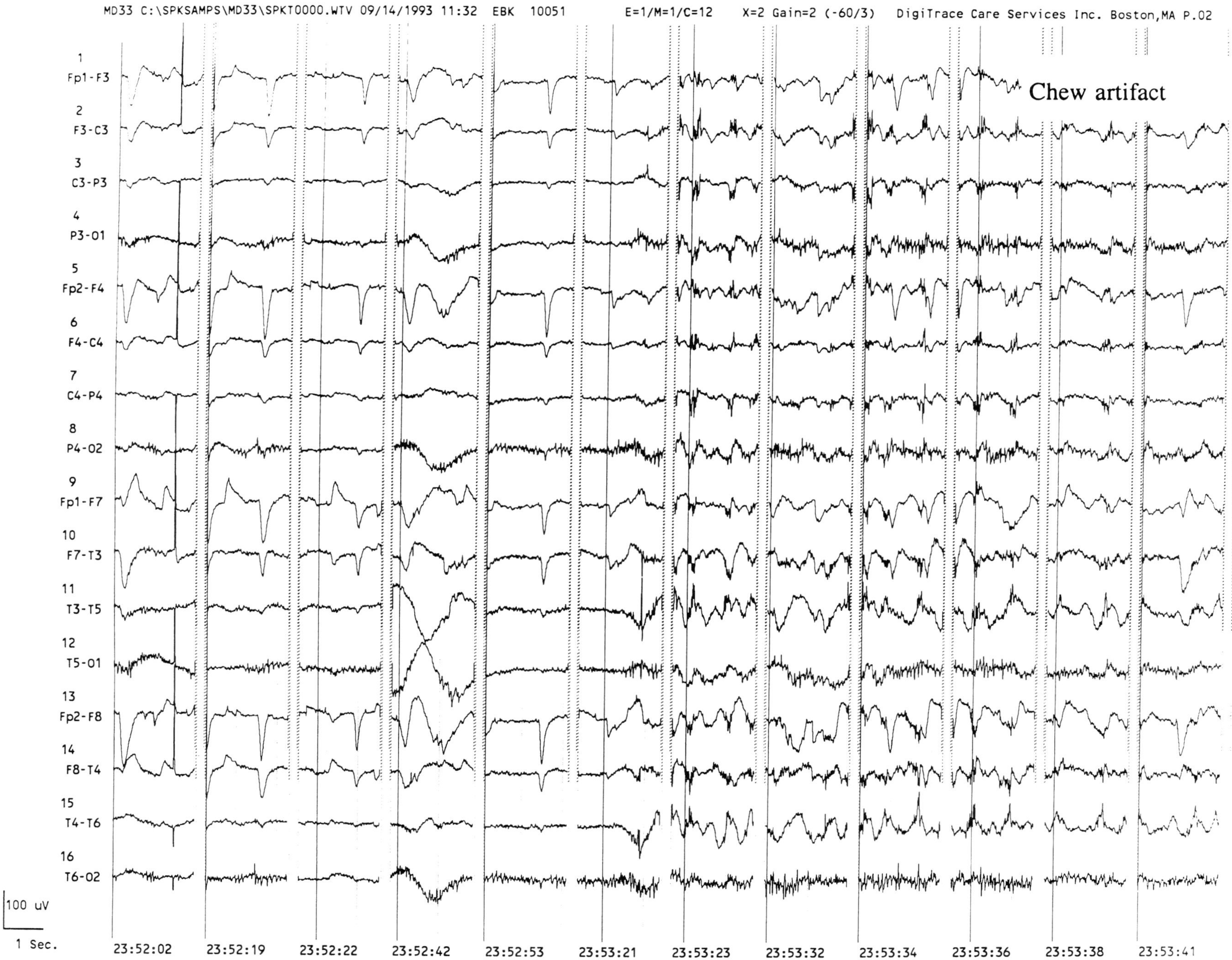
MD33 C:\SPKSAMPS\MD33\SPKT0000.WTV 09/14/1993 11:32 EBK 10051 E=1/M=1/C=12 X=2 Gain=2 (-60/3) DigiTrace Care Services Inc. Boston,MA P.02
Chew artifact
1 Fp1-F3
2 F3-C3
3 C3-P3
4 P3-O1
5 Fp2-F4
6 F4-C4
7 C4-P4
8 P4-O2
9 Fp1-F7
10 F7-T3
11 T3-T5
12 T5-O1
13 Fp2-F8
14 F8-T4
15 T4-T6
16 T6-O2
100 uV
1 Sec.
23:52:02
23:52:19
23:52:22
23:52:42
23:52:53
23:53:21
23:53:23
23:53:32
23:53:34
23:53:36
23:53:38
23:53:41

Dry Electrode Artifact

One disadvantage of ambulatory EEG monitoring is the inability of technologists to check on recording quality frequently in real time and to respond with appropriate technical adjustments as needed throughout the day, as would typically occur in an inpatient monitoring unit. Here, a dry electrode at F8 causes an artifact seen throughout this excerpt.

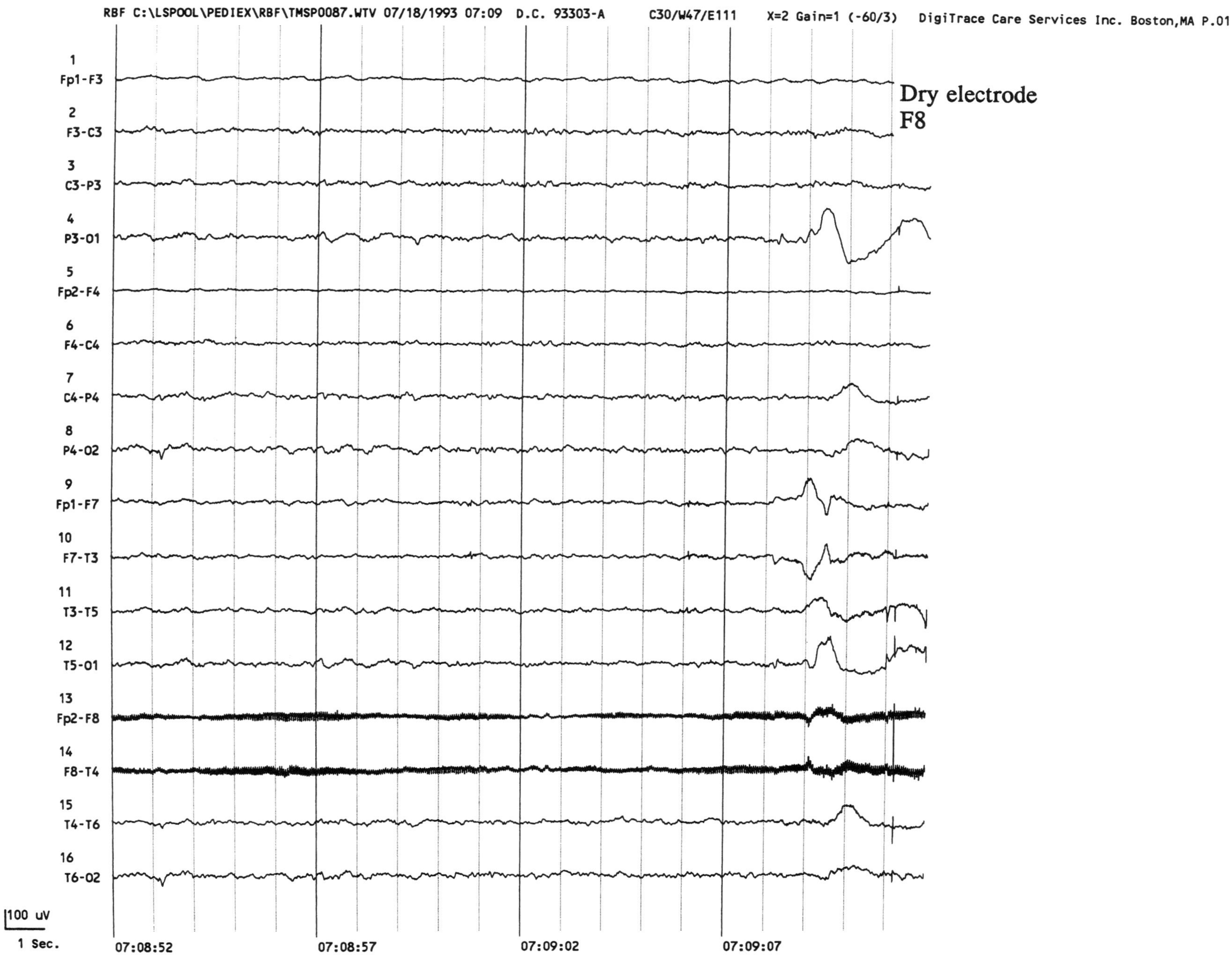
RBF C:\LSPOOL\PEDIEX\RBF\TMSP0087.WTV 07/18/1993 07:09 D.C. 93303-A C30/W47/E111 X=2 Gain=1 (-60/3) DigiTrace Care Services Inc. Boston,MA P.01
1 Fp1-F3
2 F3-C3
3 C3-P3
4 P3-O1
5 Fp2-F4
6 F4-C4
7 C4-P4
8 P4-O2
9 Fp1-F7
10 F7-T3
11 T3-T5
12 T5-O1
13 Fp2-F8
14 F8-T4
15 T4-T6
16 T6-O2
Dry electrode F8
100 uV
1 Sec.
07:08:52
07:08:57
07:09:02
07:09:07

Forehead Rubbing Artifact

As with many other patient movement artifacts, rhythmic rubbing artifact can be a potentially confusing finding on ambulatory EEG monitoring, particularly in the absence of concomitant video recording. Here, rhythmic rubbing of the forehead produces an artifact in the anterior channels, extending from the beginning of this excerpt through 20:50:16. Differentiation of such artifact from an ictal event, based on the lack of evolution of the artifact in frequency or amplitude, is critical.

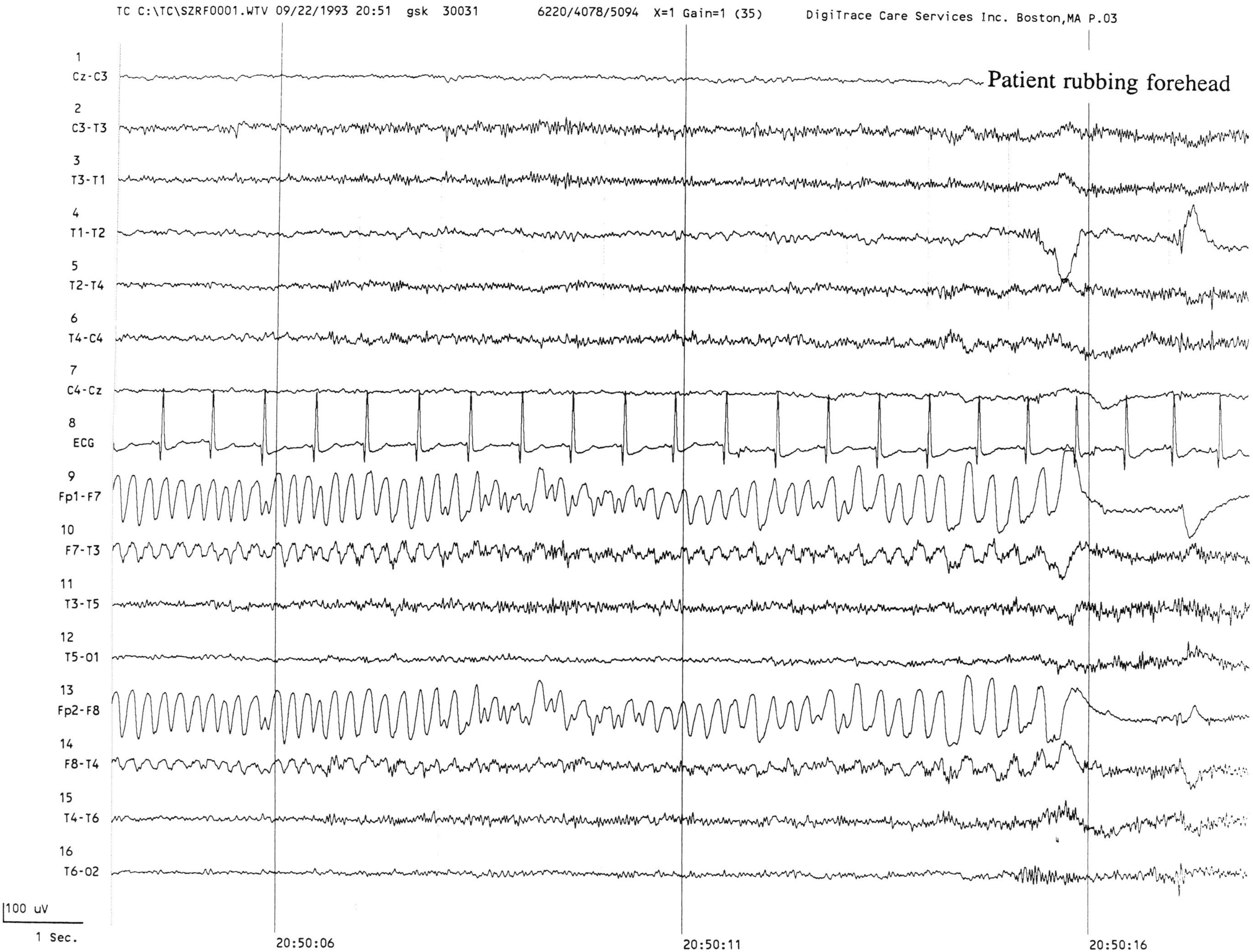
TC C:\TC\SZRF0001.WTV 09/22/1993 20:51 gsk 30031 6220/4078/5094 X=1 Gain=1 (35) DigiTrace Care Services Inc. Boston,MA P.03
Patient rubbing forehead
1 Cz-C3
2 C3-T3
3 T3-T1
4 T1-T2
5 T2-T4
6 T4-C4
7 C4-Cz
8 ECG
9 Fp1-F7
10 F7-T3
11 T3-T5
12 T5-O1
13 Fp2-F8
14 F8-T4
15 T4-T6
16 T6-O2
100 uV
1 Sec.
20:50:06
20:50:11
20:50:16

Pulse Artifact

Pulse artifact is caused by the rhythmic movement of scalp electrodes, usually over the temporal regions, by the pulsations of blood through vessels close to the skin, such as the superficial temporal artery. It is to be distinguished from the more common electrocardiographic (EKG) artifact in that pulse artifact is typically not as sharply contoured, resembles a slow wave, and follows the QRS complex rather than being simultaneous to it. Here, pulse artifact is seen in channels 9 and 10 over the left temporal region throughout this entire excerpt.

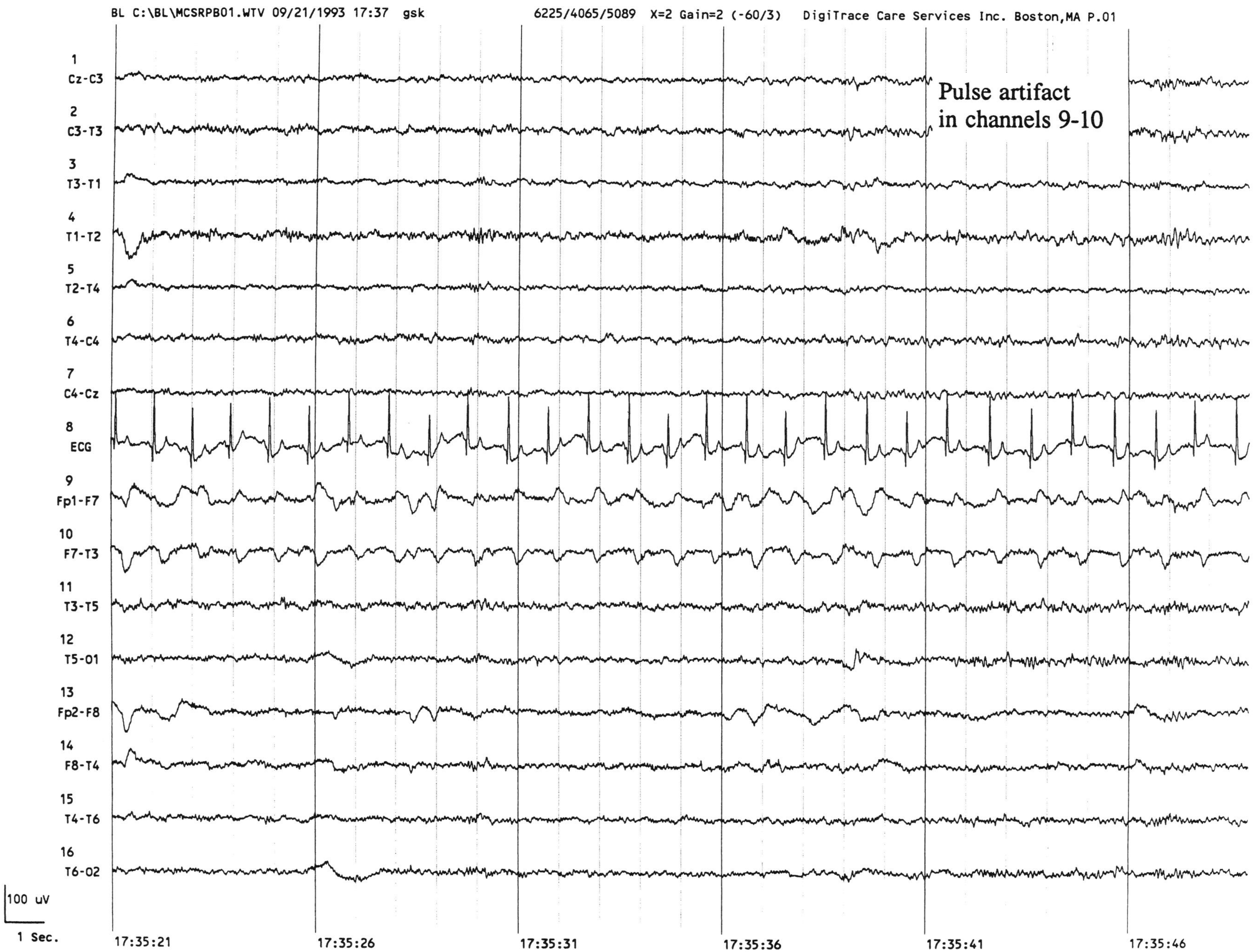
BL C:\BL\MCSRPB01.WTV 09/21/1993 17:37 gsk
6225/4065/5089 X=2 Gain=2 (-60/3)
DigiTrace Care Services Inc. Boston,MA P.01
1 Cz-C3
2 C3-T3
3 T3-T1
4 T1-T2
5 T2-T4
6 T4-C4
7 C4-Cz
8 ECG
9 Fp1-F7
10 F7-T3
11 T3-T5
12 T5-O1
13 Fp2-F8
14 F8-T4
15 T4-T6
16 T6-O2
100 uV
1 Sec.
17:35:21
17:35:26
17:35:31
17:35:36
17:35:41
17:35:46
Pulse artifact in channels 9-10

ABNORMAL EPILEPTIFORM ACTIVITY

Focal Mesial Temporal Spikes Recorded by Spike Detection Algorithm

Six separate files captured by the spike detection algorithm demonstrate focal spikes with phase reversal at the right sphenoidal electrode (Sp2). With scalp electrodes only, the epileptiform discharges would have been far less obvious (see channels 13 and 14).

MA40M C:\MA40M\SPKT0000.WTV 06/06/1992 20:30 jxg ************* e=d, m=42, c=3 X=1 Gain=2 (-60/3) DigiTrace Care Services Inc. Boston,MA P.04

Spike Detection File
2 Seconds Per File
12 Files/Page

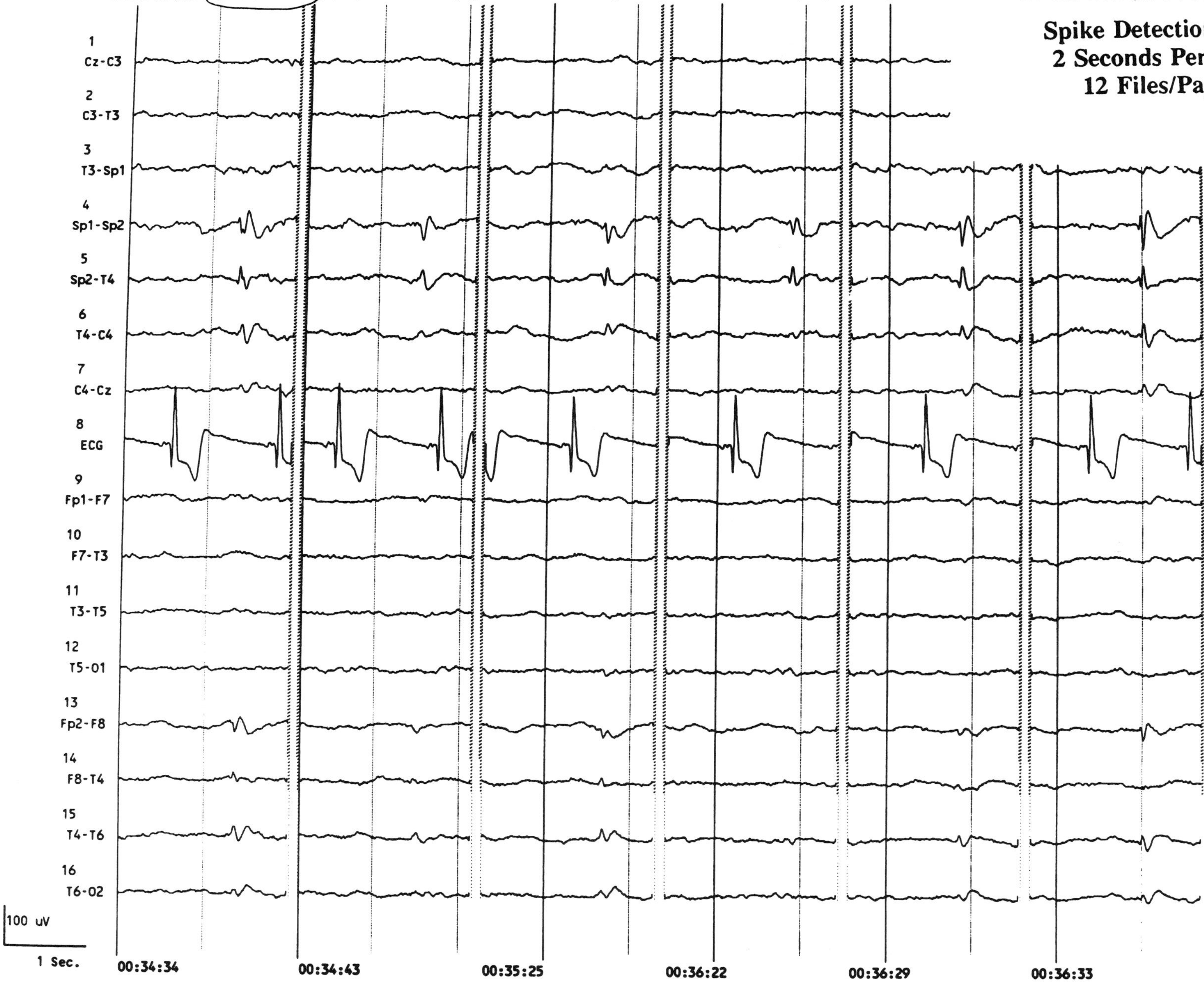

EPILEPTIFORM 2

Focal Anterior Temporal Spikes Recorded by Spike Detection Algorithm

Multiple spikes are captured in these files, phase-reversing at the T1 and F7 electrodes. All of these epileptiform discharges were seen during sleep and had not been present on a routine EEG recording.

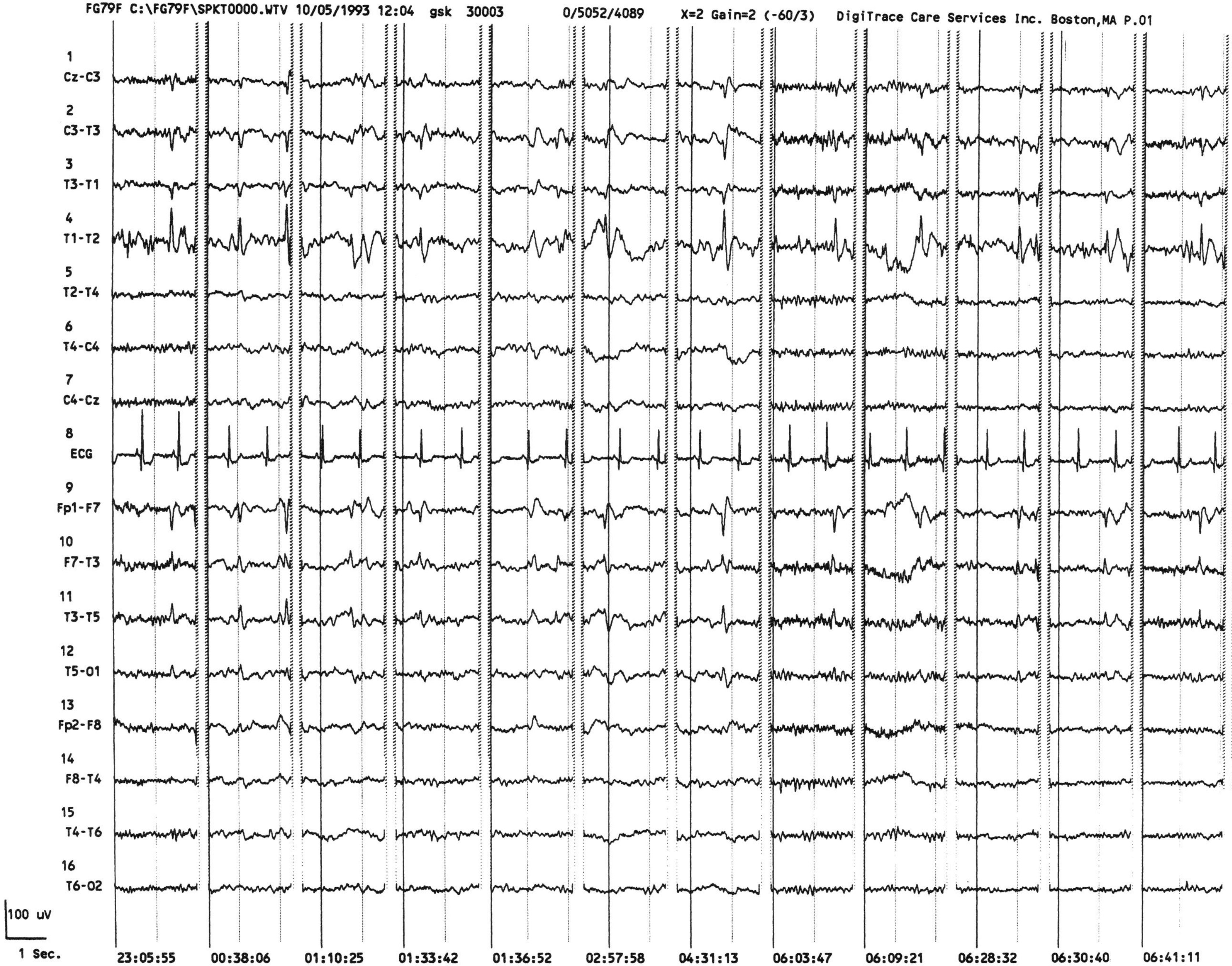
FG79F C:\FG79F\SPKT0000.WTV 10/05/1993 12:04 gsk 30003 0/5052/4089 X=2 Gain=2 (-60/3) DigiTrace Care Services Inc. Boston,MA P.01
1 Cz-C3
2 C3-T3
3 T3-T1
4 T1-T2
5 T2-T4
6 T4-C4
7 C4-Cz
8 ECG
9 Fp1-F7
10 F7-T3
11 T3-T5
12 T5-01
13 Fp2-F8
14 F8-T4
15 T4-T6
16 T6-02
100 uV
1 Sec.
23:05:55
00:38:06
01:10:25
01:33:42
01:36:52
02:57:58
04:31:13
06:03:47
06:09:21
06:28:32
06:30:40
06:41:11

Bifrontal Spike-Wave Complexes Recorded by Spike Detection Algorithm

In this excerpt, frequent bifrontal spike-wave discharges are captured by the spike detection algorithm, with several files recorded here within just a few minutes' time.

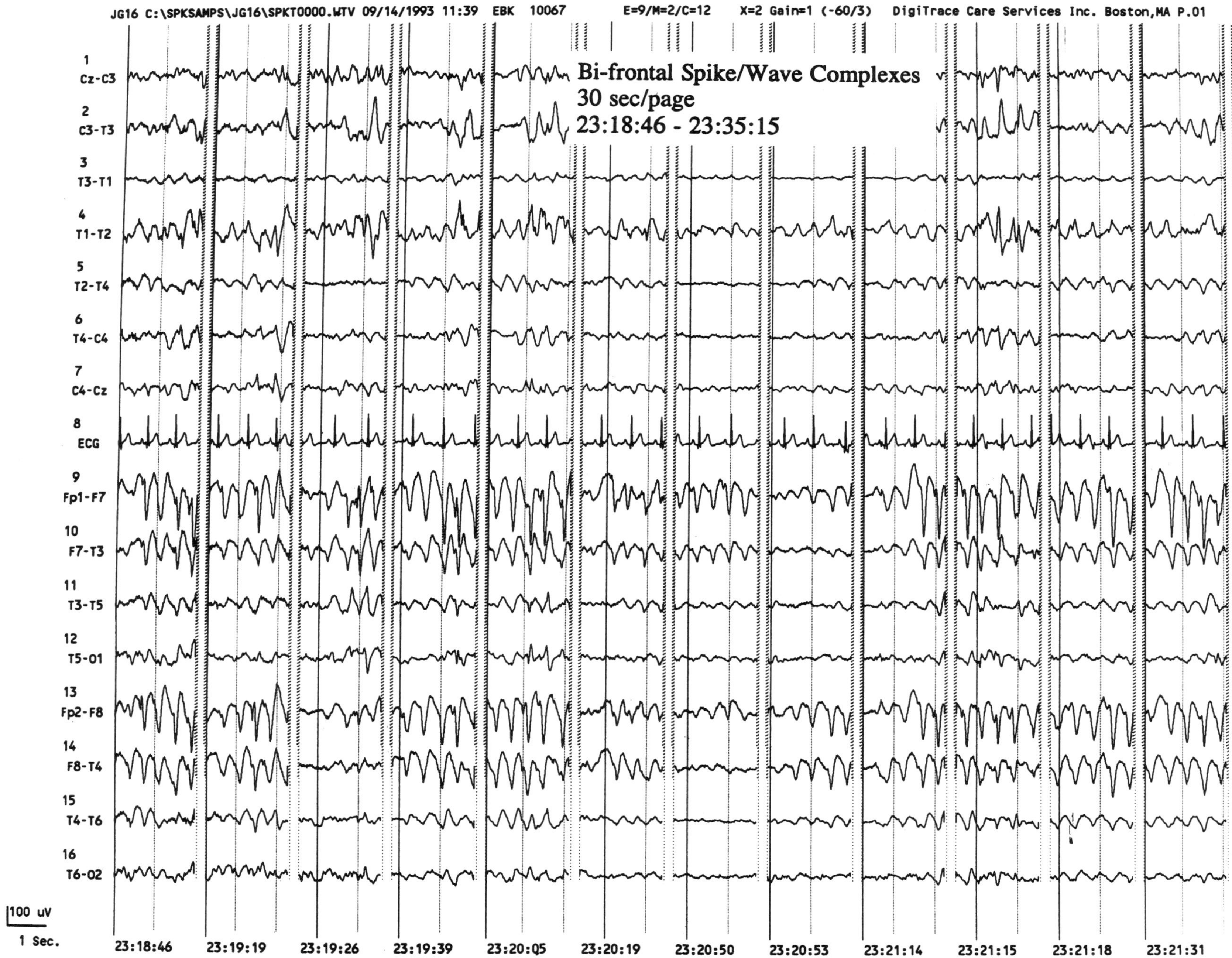
JG16 C:\SPKSAMPS\JG16\SPKT0000.WTV 09/14/1993 11:39 EBK 10067 E=9/M=2/C=12 X=2 Gain=1 (-60/3) DigiTrace Care Services Inc. Boston,MA P.01
Bi-frontal Spike/Wave Complexes
30 sec/page
23:18:46 - 23:35:15
1 Cz-C3
2 C3-T3
3 T3-T1
4 T1-T2
5 T2-T4
6 T4-C4
7 C4-Cz
8 ECG
9 Fp1-F7
10 F7-T3
11 T3-T5
12 T5-O1
13 Fp2-F8
14 F8-T4
15 T4-T6
16 T6-O2
100 uV
1 Sec.
23:18:46
23:19:19
23:19:26
23:19:39
23:20:05
23:20:19
23:20:50
23:20:53
23:21:14
23:21:15
23:21:18
23:21:31

EPILEPTIFORM 4

Rolandic Spikes

In this excerpt, several independent bilateral centrotemporal (Rolandic) spikes can be seen phase-reversing at the C3 and C4 electrodes. In the same channels, a sleep spindle is seen beginning at 04:25:08.

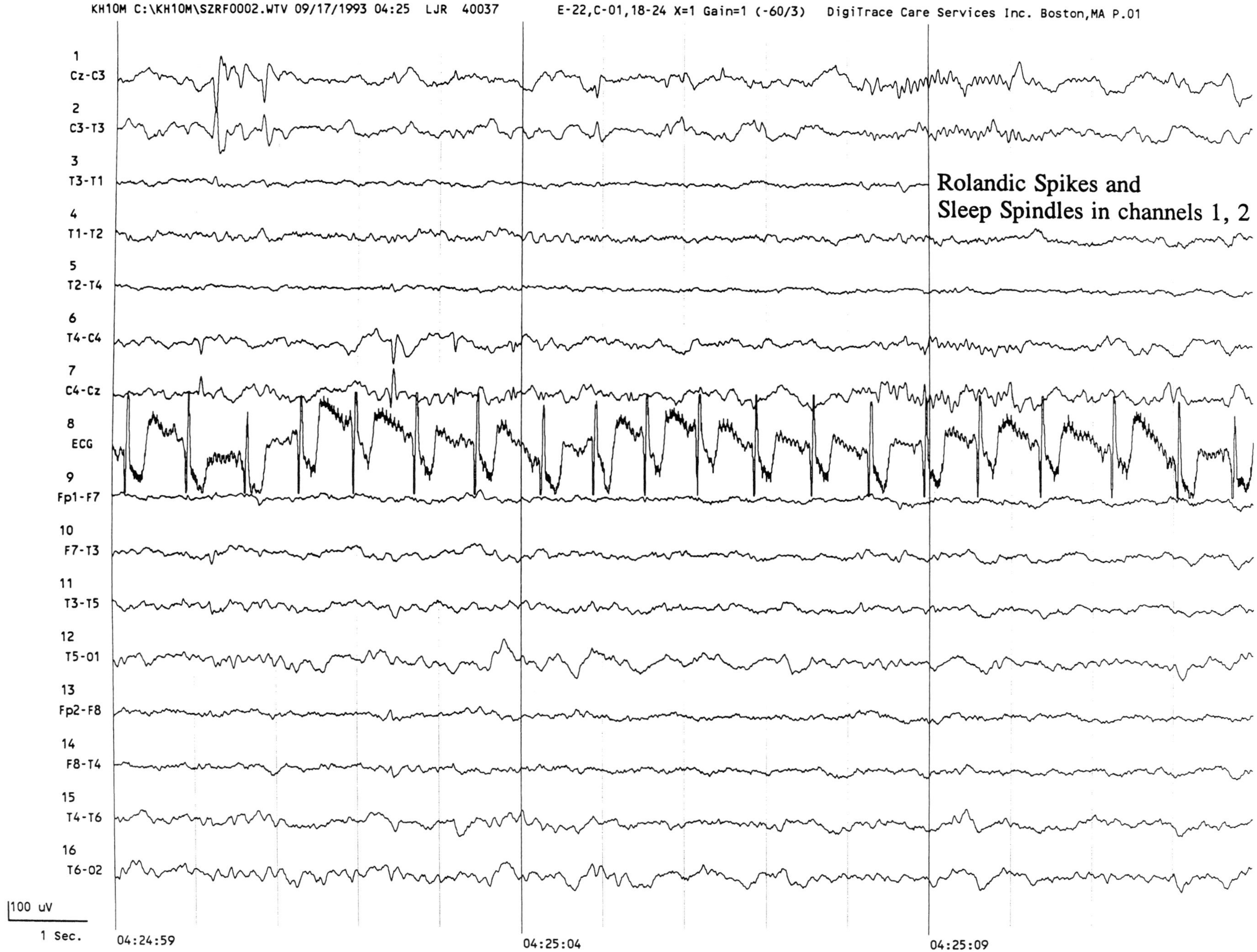

Rolandic Spikes and
Sleep Spindles in channels 1, 2

3-Per-Second Spike-and-Wave Activity Recorded by Spike Detection Algorithm

The third and fourth files on this page demonstrate generalized spike-and-slow-wave activity recurring at about a 3-per-second frequency.

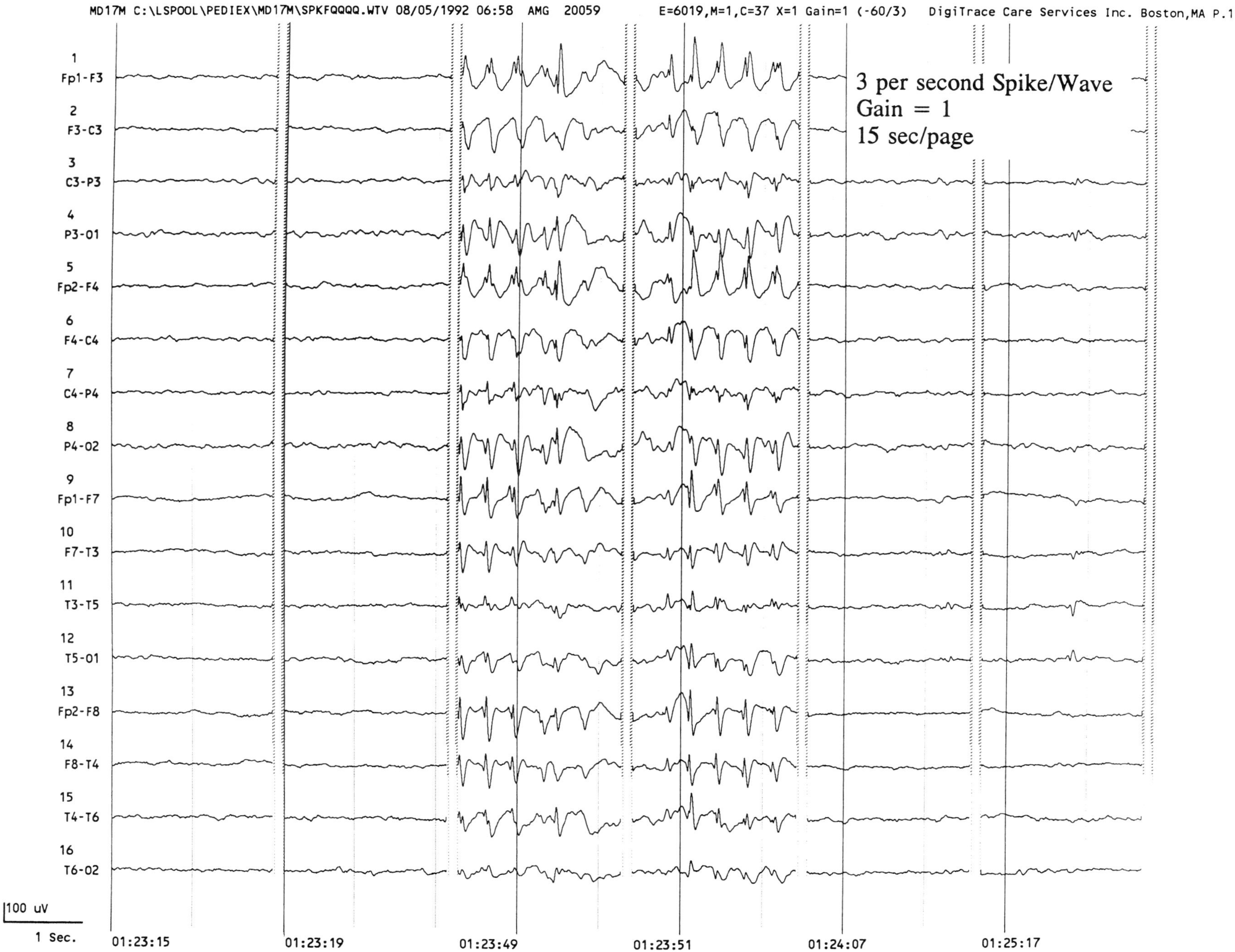
MD17M C:\LSPOOL\PEDIEX\MD17M\SPKFQQQQ.WTV 08/05/1992 06:58 AMG 20059 E=6019,M=1,C=37 X=1 Gain=1 (-60/3) DigiTrace Care Services Inc. Boston,MA P.11
3 per second Spike/Wave
Gain = 1
15 sec/page
1 Fp1-F3
2 F3-C3
3 C3-P3
4 P3-O1
5 Fp2-F4
6 F4-C4
7 C4-P4
8 P4-O2
9 Fp1-F7
10 F7-T3
11 T3-T5
12 T5-O1
13 Fp2-F8
14 F8-T4
15 T4-T6
16 T6-O2
100 uV
1 Sec.
01:23:15
01:23:19
01:23:49
01:23:51
01:24:07
01:25:17

Generalized Spike-and-Wave Activity Recorded by Seizure Detection Algorithm (Page 1 of 2)

The onset of generalized spike-and-slow wave activity is captured by the seizure detection algorithm in this excerpt. At 13:20:15 the epileptiform activity begins at about a 3-per-second frequency. The tracing continues on the next page.

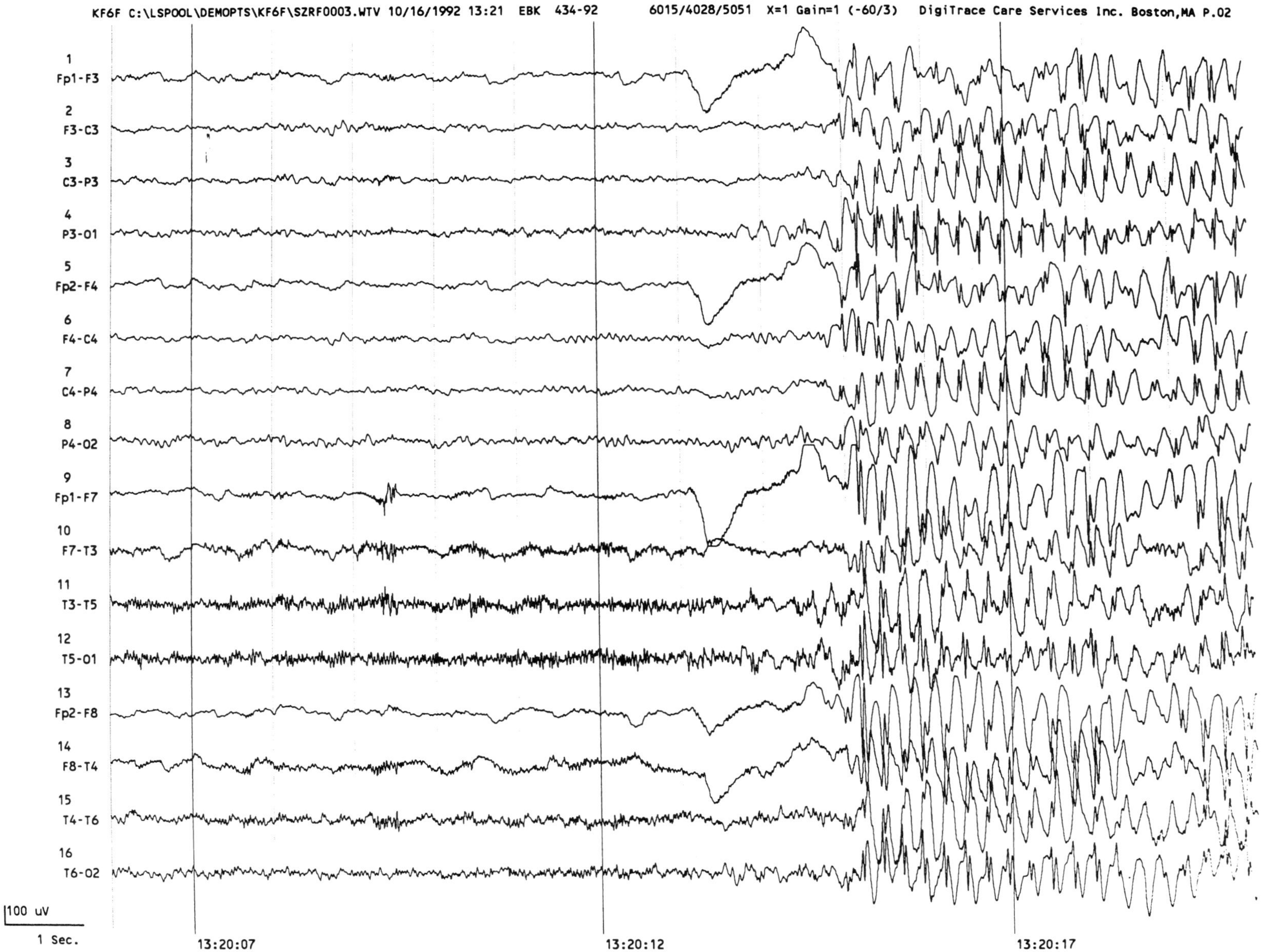
KF6F C:\LSPOOL\DEMOPTS\KF6F\SZRF0003.WTV 10/16/1992 13:21 EBK 434-92
6015/4028/5051 X=1 Gain=1 (-60/3) DigiTrace Care Services Inc. Boston,MA P.02
1 Fp1-F3
2 F3-C3
3 C3-P3
4 P3-O1
5 Fp2-F4
6 F4-C4
7 C4-P4
8 P4-O2
9 Fp1-F7
10 F7-T3
11 T3-T5
12 T5-O1
13 Fp2-F8
14 F8-T4
15 T4-T6
16 T6-O2
100 uV
1 Sec.
13:20:07
13:20:12
13:20:17

Generalized Spike-and-Wave Activity Recorded by Seizure Detection Algorithm (Page 2 of 2)

Generalized epileptiform activity continues in this excerpt, with a gradual diminution of activity over 2 seconds (13:20:27 to 13:20:29) before some background disorganization and slowing are seen postictally. The total duration of the epileptiform activity is about 15 seconds.

KF6F C:\LSPOOL\DEMOPTS\KF6F\SZRF0003.WTV 10/16/1992 13:21 EBK 434-92 6015/4028/5051 X=1 Gain=1 (-60/3) DigiTrace Care Services Inc. Boston,MA P.03

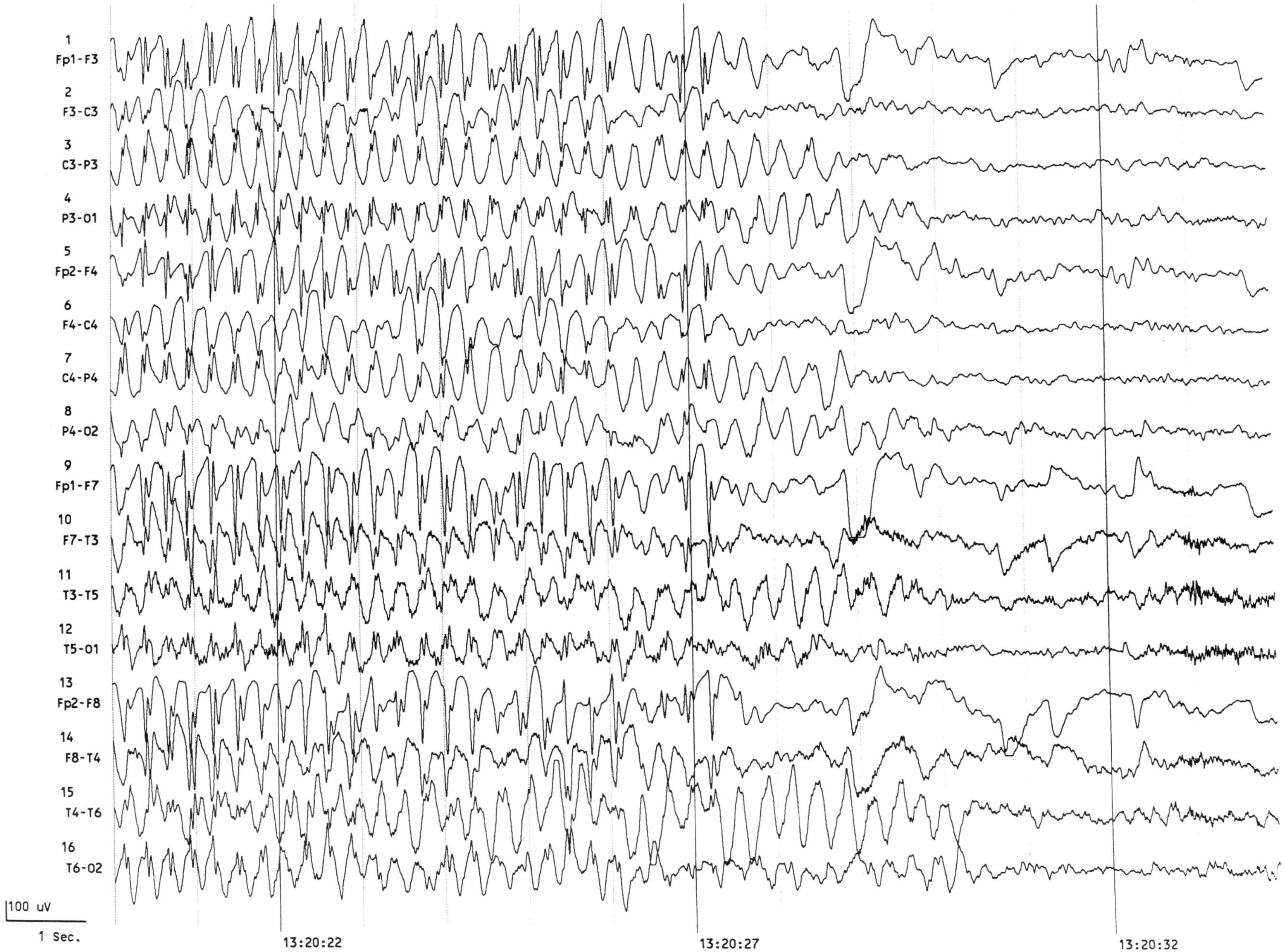

EPILEPTIFORM 7

Brief Generalized Spike-and-Wave Activity Recorded by Seizure Detection Algorithm

An 8-second period of epileptiform activity was captured by the seizure detection algorithm. At onset (21:39:46), the activity appears frontocentral in localization but quickly spreads over 1 to 2 seconds to become more generalized in distribution. The 2.5- to 3-per-second activity, which includes some polyspike discharges, terminates fairly abruptly at 21:39:54.

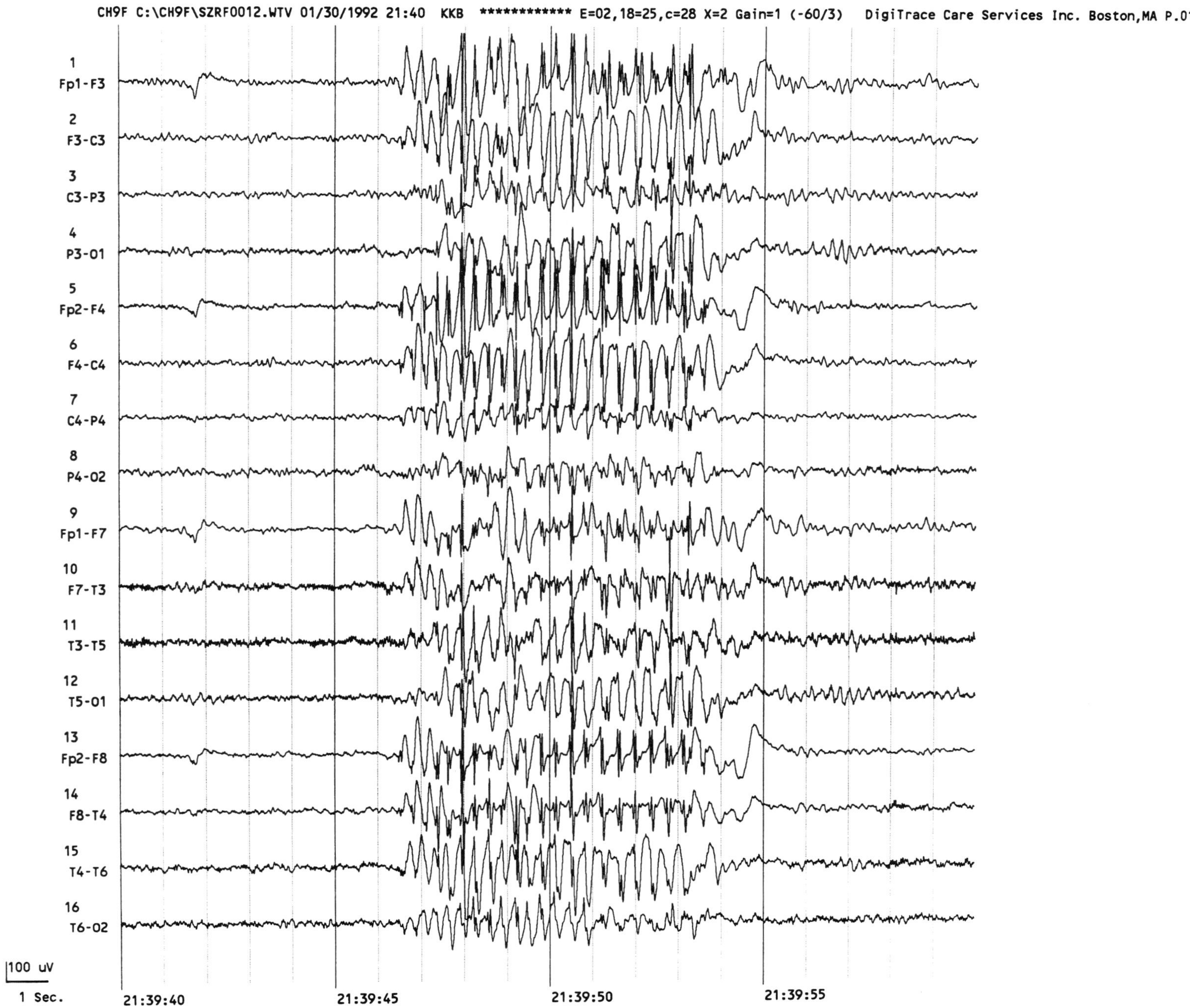
CH9F C:\CH9F\SZRF0012.WTV 01/30/1992 21:40 KKB ************* E=02,18=25,c=28 X=2 Gain=1 (-60/3) DigiTrace Care Services Inc. Boston,MA P.01
1 Fp1-F3
2 F3-C3
3 C3-P3
4 P3-O1
5 Fp2-F4
6 F4-C4
7 C4-P4
8 P4-O2
9 Fp1-F7
10 F7-T3
11 T3-T5
12 T5-O1
13 Fp2-F8
14 F8-T4
15 T4-T6
16 T6-O2
100 uV
1 Sec.
21:39:40
21:39:45
21:39:50
21:39:55

Left Frontotemporal Seizure Recorded by Pushbutton Activation (Page 1 of 2)

This seizure was recorded after the patient activated the waist-worn event button to indicate the occurrence of typical symptoms. The onset of this seizure is at about 8:49:22, with low-voltage fast activity seen broadly across the left frontotemporal region (in channels 2–4 and 9–11). The tracing continues on the next page.

FG79F C:\FG79F\MCSRPB01.WTV 06/24/1993 08:49 gsk 0/5052/4089 X=2 Gain=2 (-60/3) DigiTrace Care Services Inc. Boston,MA P.04

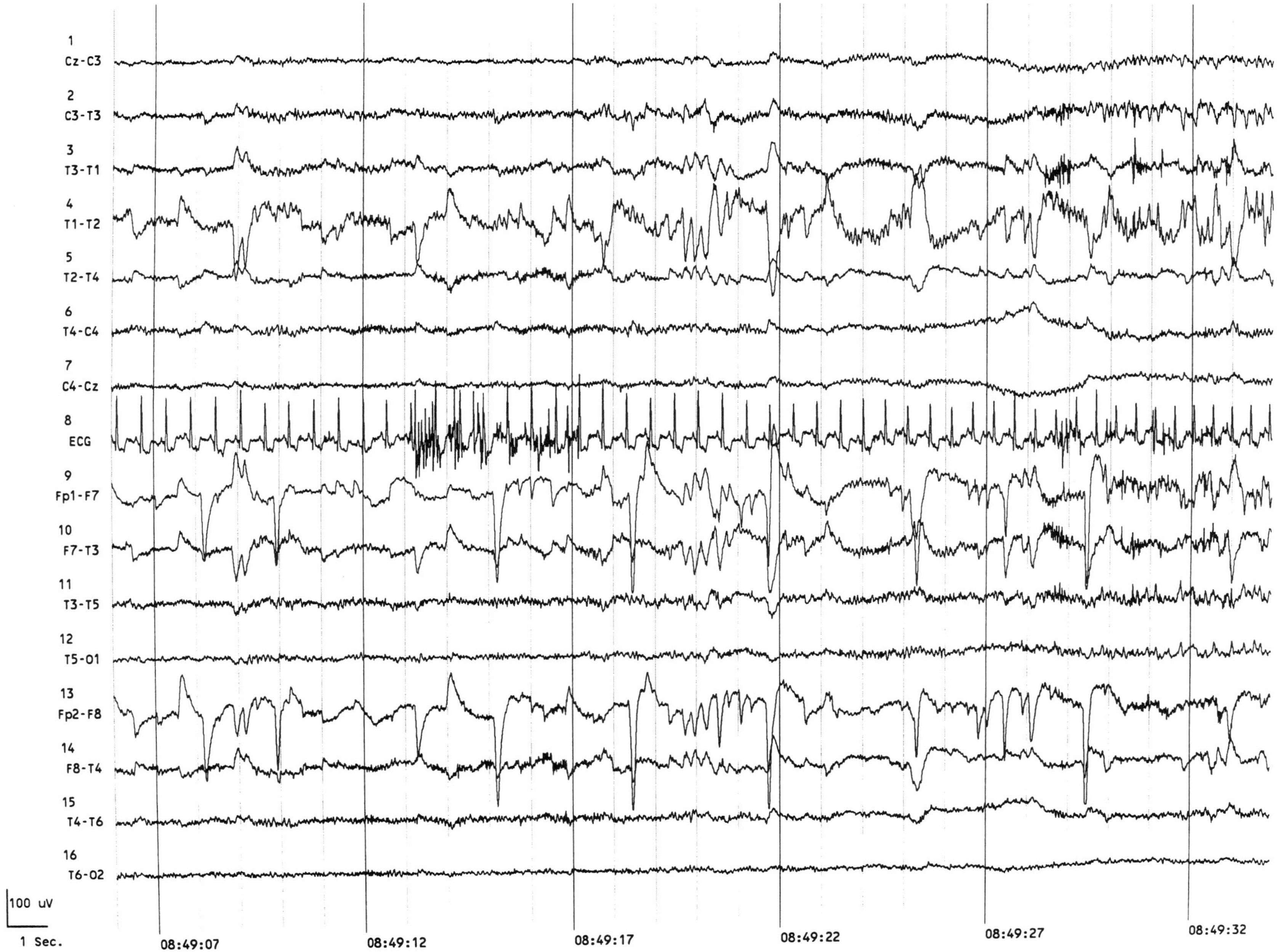

Left Frontotemporal Seizure Recorded by Pushbutton Activation (Page 2 of 2)

The focal epileptiform activity that began on the previous page evolves here to include rhythmic higher voltage sharp activity initially occurring at a 3-per-second frequency, tapering down to 1 per second, and eventually terminating at about 08:49:51. The artifact created by the pushbutton activation is present at 08:49:42.

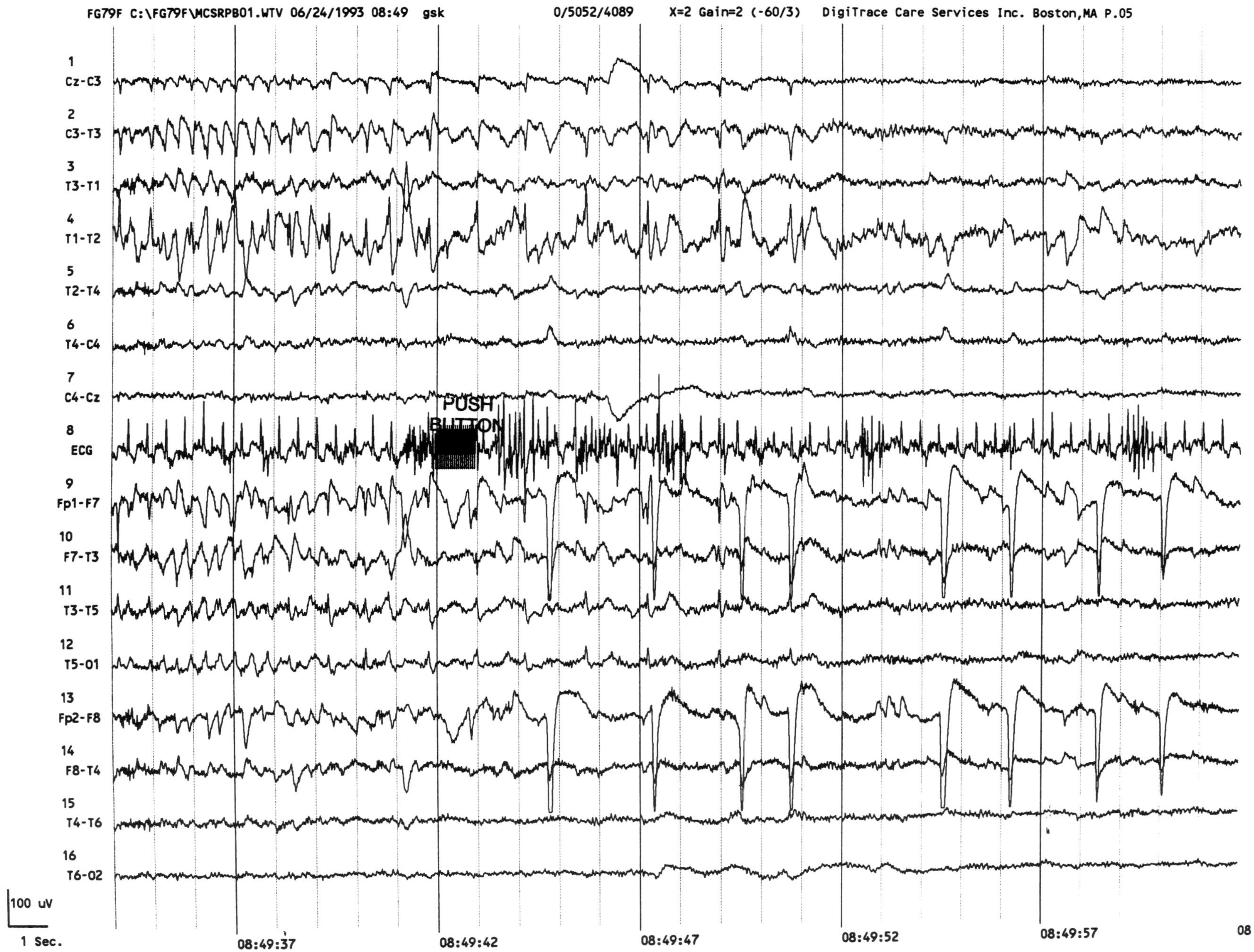
FG79F C:\FG79F\MCSRPB01.WTV 06/24/1993 08:49 gsk
0/5052/4089
X=2 Gain=2 (-60/3)
DigiTrace Care Services Inc. Boston,MA P.05
1 Cz-C3
2 C3-T3
3 T3-T1
4 T1-T2
5 T2-T4
6 T4-C4
7 C4-Cz
8 ECG
9 Fp1-F7
10 F7-T3
11 T3-T5
12 T5-O1
13 Fp2-F8
14 F8-T4
15 T4-T6
16 T6-O2
PUSH BUTTON
100 uV
1 Sec.
08:49:37
08:49:42
08:49:47
08:49:52
08:49:57
08

Frontal Onset Epileptiform Activity Recorded by Seizure Detection Algorithm

This file was captured by the seizure detection algorithm from the same patient recorded in the prior figure. Preceding the more generalized epileptiform activity, an isolated spike-and-slow-wave discharge that is bifrontal but more evident in the left frontal region is seen at 03:48:10.

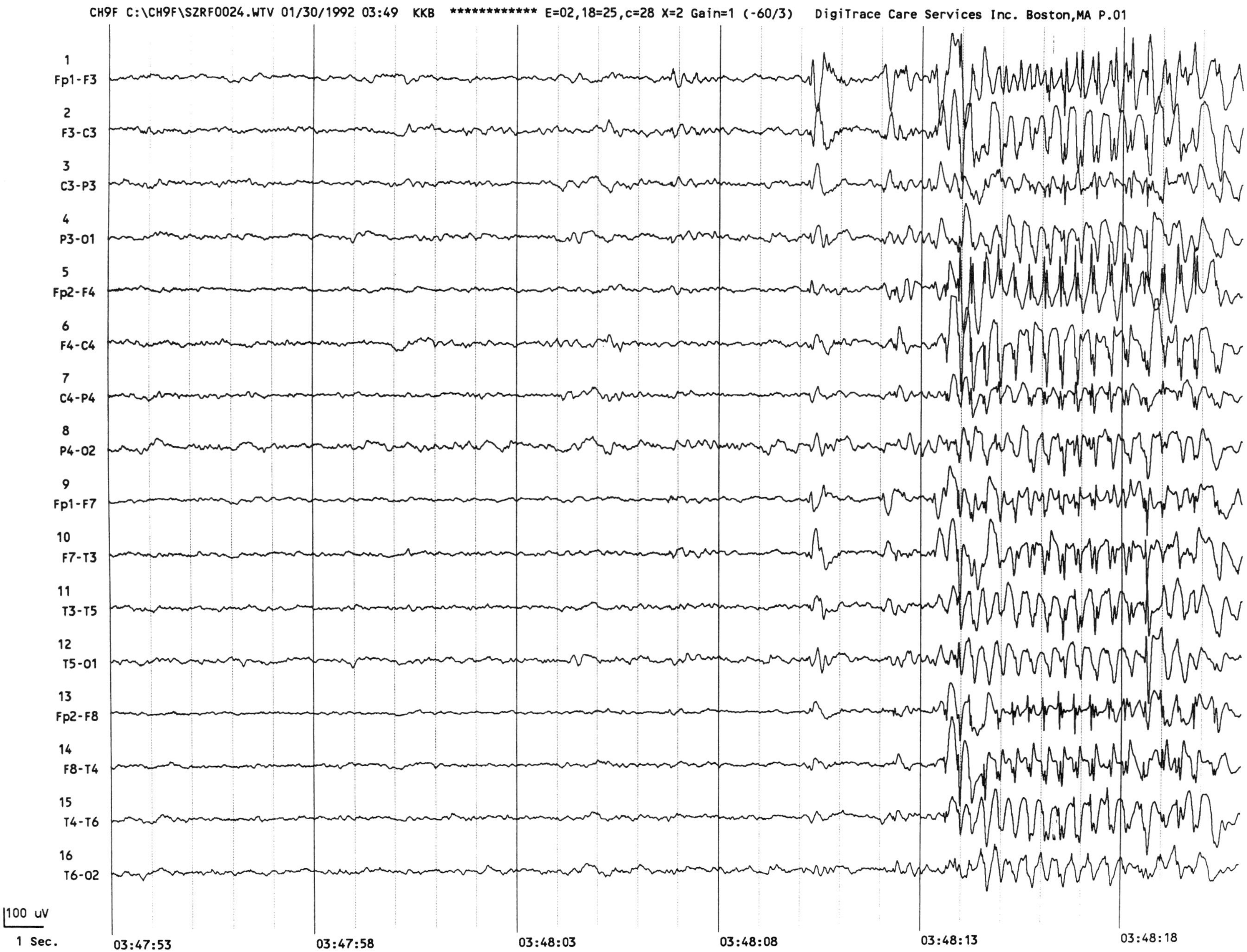
CH9F C:\CH9F\SZRF0024.WTV 01/30/1992 03:49 KKB ************* E=02,18=25,c=28 X=2 Gain=1 (-60/3) DigiTrace Care Services Inc. Boston,MA P.01
1 Fp1-F3
2 F3-C3
3 C3-P3
4 P3-O1
5 Fp2-F4
6 F4-C4
7 C4-P4
8 P4-O2
9 Fp1-F7
10 F7-T3
11 T3-T5
12 T5-O1
13 Fp2-F8
14 F8-T4
15 T4-T6
16 T6-O2
100 uV
1 Sec.
03:47:53
03:47:58
03:48:03
03:48:08
03:48:13
03:48:18

Right Mesial Temporal Seizure Recorded by Pushbutton Activation (Page 1 of 2)

A clinically symptomatic event prompted the pushbutton activation at 17:30:16 on this two-page excerpt. About 6 seconds prior, rhythmic theta-frequency activity begins in the right temporal region, phase-reversing at the right sphenoidal electrode (Sp2). This activity evolves over the next 5 to 10 seconds and becomes obscured by muscle artifact. The tracing continues on the next page.

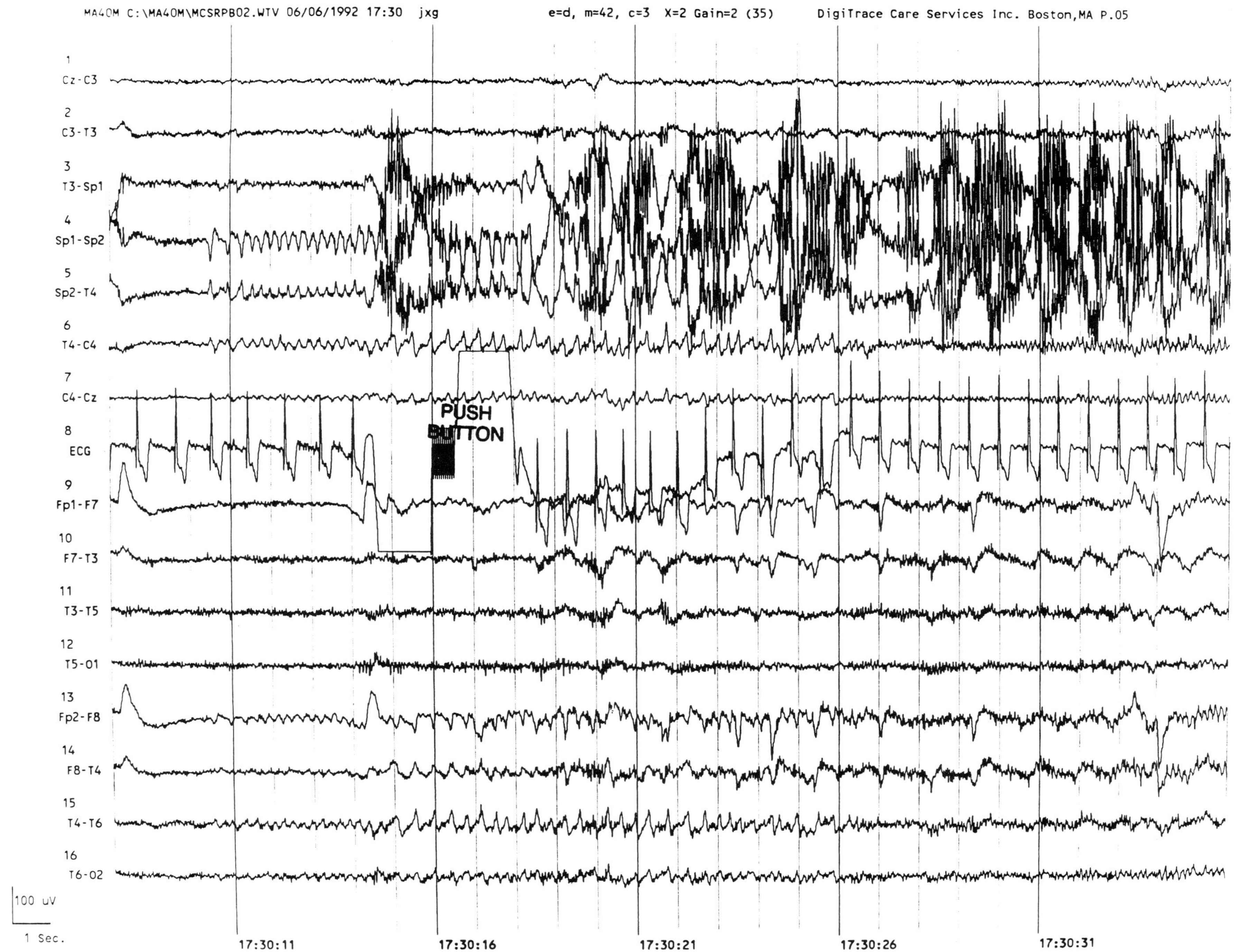
MA40M C:\MA40M\MCSRPB02.WTV 06/06/1992 17:30 jxg
e=d, m=42, c=3 X=2 Gain=2 (35)
DigiTrace Care Services Inc. Boston,MA P.05
1 Cz-C3
2 C3-T3
3 T3-Sp1
4 Sp1-Sp2
5 Sp2-T4
6 T4-C4
7 C4-Cz
8 ECG
9 Fp1-F7
10 F7-T3
11 T3-T5
12 T5-O1
13 Fp2-F8
14 F8-T4
15 T4-T6
16 T6-O2
PUSH BUTTON
100 uV
1 Sec.
17:30:11
17:30:16
17:30:21
17:30:26
17:30:31

Right Mesial Temporal Seizure Recorded by Pushbutton Activation (Page 2 of 2)

As the seizure beginning on the previous page progresses further, spread of the epileptiform activity to the left temporal and central regions becomes apparent by 17:30:37.

MA40M C:\MA40M\MCSRPB02.WTV 06/06/1992 17:30 jxg e=d, m=42, c=3 X=2 Gain=2 (35) DigiTrace Care Services Inc. Boston,MA P.05

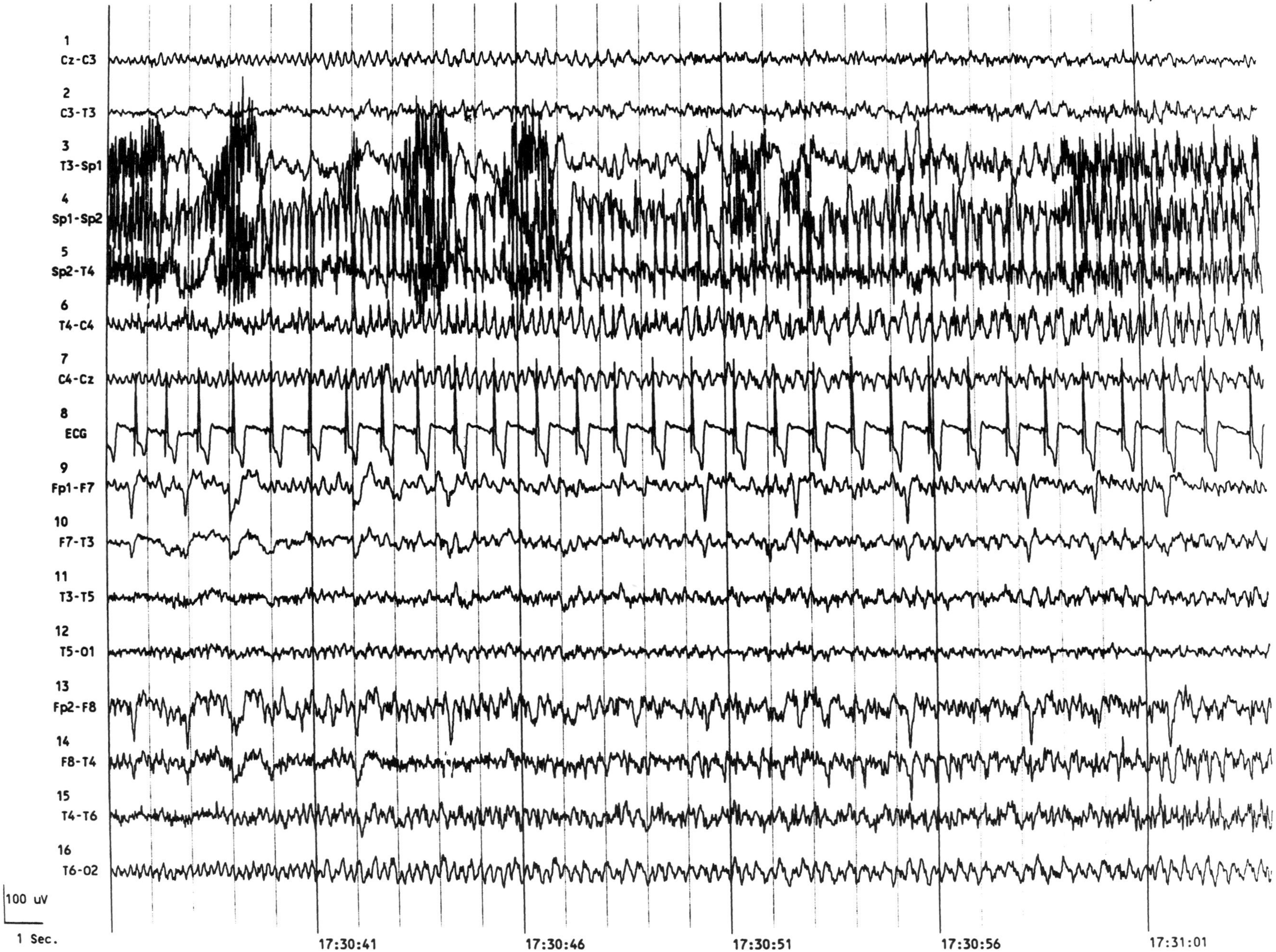

EPILEPTIFORM 11

Frontal Seizure Recorded by Pushbutton Activation

The pushbutton activation is noted at 19:51:41. About 2 seconds prior, rhythmic delta-frequency activity in bilateral frontal regions is seen, with a progression to sharp-and-slow-wave complexes with 2- to 2.5-per-second frequency over both frontocentral regions. Courtesy Edward H. Kovnar, MD.

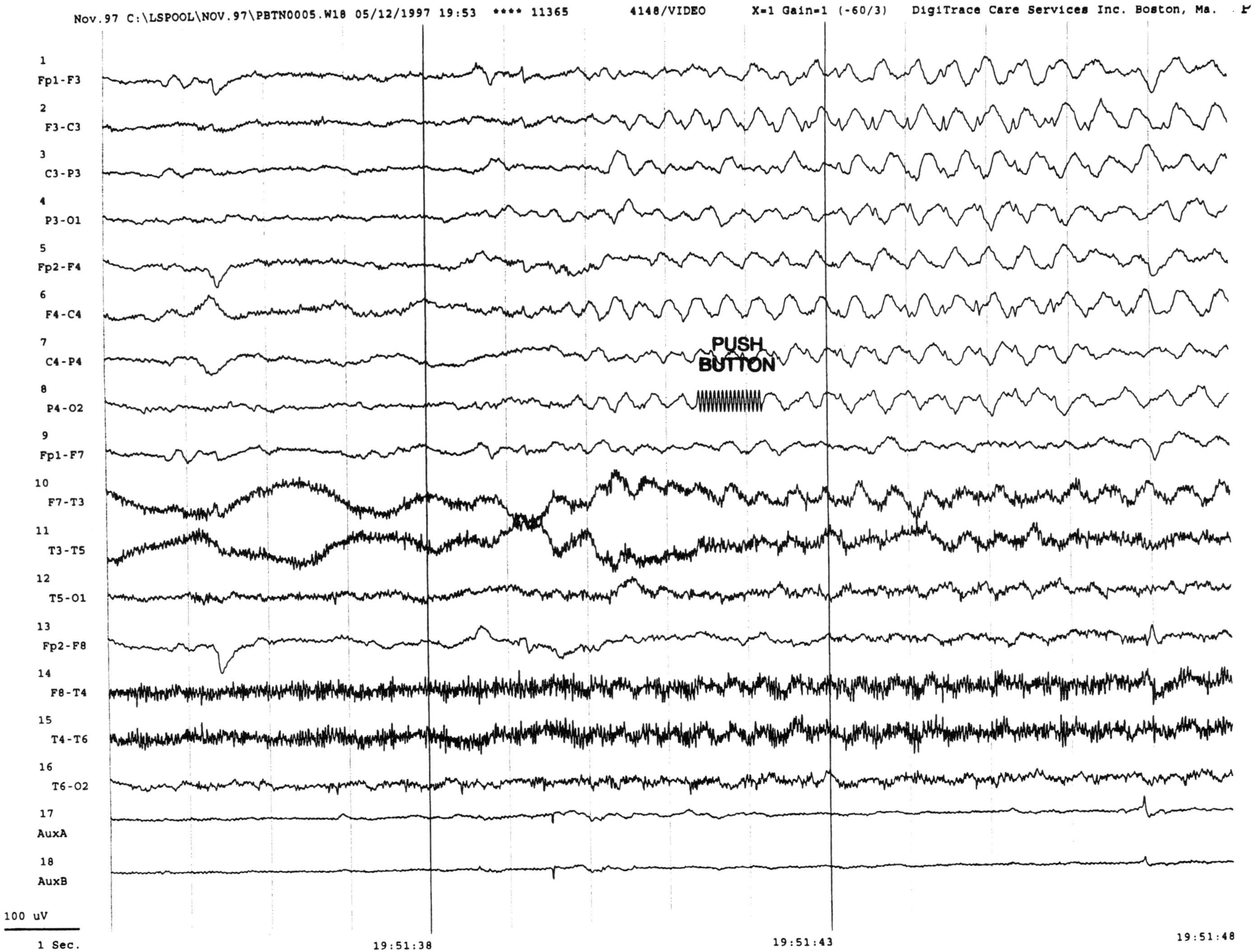
Nov.97 C:\LSPOOL\NOV.97\PBTN0005.W18 05/12/1997 19:53 **** 11365
4148/VIDEO
X=1 Gain=1 (-60/3)
DigiTrace Care Services Inc. Boston, Ma.
1 Fp1-F3
2 F3-C3
3 C3-P3
4 P3-O1
5 Fp2-F4
6 F4-C4
7 C4-P4
8 P4-O2
9 Fp1-F7
10 F7-T3
11 T3-T5
12 T5-O1
13 Fp2-F8
14 F8-T4
15 T4-T6
16 T6-O2
17 AuxA
18 AuxB
PUSH BUTTON
100 uV
1 Sec.
19:51:38
19:51:43
19:51:48

Index